"I loved *Great Body No Diet* and especially the chapter on the importance of water for health, including weight loss. In simple words, I have found knowledge I have been waiting for all my life."

- Margaret Anderson, Co-Author of *What Can You Do To Help Our World?*

"This book contains a simple yet profound approach to health and well being that focuses on a heightened sense of body consciousness. It offers the reader a refreshing alternative to the extreme and unnatural diets out there by weaving in principles of healthy living that are not only painless but also highly logical and aimed at finding and enhancing pleasure in our daily lives. I strongly recommend this book to anyone who would like to obtain a happier and healthier quotidian."

- Keala Carter, AFAA Certified Personal Trainer and Holistic Nutritionist.

"Easy to read, down-to-earth, and full of helpful advice. I recommend that everyone read this book. It is a one-on-one experience of writer to reader. No finger pointing. Only positive thoughts."

- Barbara Wolf, Founder of *Global Meditations Network* and Co-Author of *What Can You Do To Help Our World?*

"The premise of *Great Body No Diet* is simple, and speaks greatly on how to be healthy and balanced without sacrificing foods you crave. It addresses way more than diet and eating, to include fitness, meditation and overall well being. It offers fantastic information on what to avoid in life for better overall health. Written in an engaging, clever and story telling way! A must have!"

- Samar Younes, Visual Director of Creative Development, Coach

"I have battled with weight loss for most of my life namely because of *conventional* diets that never worked for the long hall! After adopting Racha's practical and easy tips, I managed to get a grip on my unhealthy relationship with food. If I could summarize this book into one statement I would say it is about a fit woman with a beautiful body sharing her secrets on how she manages to stay so slim while eating whatever she *feels* like eating! Thank you for your generosity dear Racha and for helping me to finally make peace with food!"

- Rouba Zeidan, Singer/Songwriter & Communication Specialist

# GREAT BODY
# NO DIET

*Practical Solutions for Reaching Your Ideal Weight
and Maintaining It for Life*

———

**Racha Zeidan**

**Mangosteen Publishing**
Charlottesville, Virginia 22903, USA
info@mangosteenpublishing.com
www.mangosteenpublishing.com

Published in 2013
**Editing, Design and Print by CreateSpace, an Amazon Company**
Location: 7290 B. Investment Drive, Charleston, SC 29418 USA

ISBN: 0988290502
ISBN-13: 978-0-9882905-0-1
Library of Congress Control Number: 2012916401

**Purchase bulk orders online at a discounted rate by visiting
www.greatbodynodiet.com.**

# CONTENTS

# PREFACE

Two experiences prompted me to start this book.

One was when I began to notice how often people complain after a meal about how much they ate. Comments like, "I've gained so much weight"; "I can't believe I just ate all that food"; "Do you know how fattening this dessert is?"; or "Do you know how many calories are in this meal we just ate?" spoiled the atmosphere for everyone at the table and led to friends and family resenting food instead of appreciating it.

I was getting fed up with this type of post-meal conversation, because to me, food is not fattening; it is a blessing. When I have the chance to eat something sweet, I see it as a positive treat because I love sweets and they give me energy. Though I was irritated by such comments, I could totally understand the fear, uncertainty, and guilt that lots of people have these days when it comes to eating. I used to have it too, but not anymore. My hope is that this book will help change readers' relationship with and attitude toward food.

The second and more personal reason I started this project was because people kept asking me the same questions: "How come you eat anything you like and stay slim?", "How are you in control of your weight?".

I too became curious and wanted to understand why I was slim, knowing for sure that I was not following a diet or a strict workout schedule and that I had gained weight several times in the past, lost it all, and remained on the slim side. So in 2006, I decided to write an email and send it to my friends, telling them about my diet-free eating habits and moderate fitness lifestyle. I began recording my thoughts, habits, and actions. With time and lots of observation of my behavior, I discovered that I *was* following a certain method that resulted in a great body for life.

As the knowledge accumulated, the e-mail grew, and I continued writing, experimenting and researching in my free time over the course of seven years. Here I am today, proud to share with you practical solutions for reaching your ideal weight and maintaining it for life, in a diet-free and guilt-free way.

Do not assume "Great Body No Diet" advocates that you can eat whatever you want in large quantities and whenever you want it, without gaining weight. This book promotes eating well and from all food types, explains how and when to eat and drink without having to use a calorie calculator and without having to worry each time you feel like chocolate cake. Food will become the last thing on your mind, and you will be fearless, in control and strong on the inside.

# DISCLAIMER

This book is for people who are above 21 years of age.

If you are happy with your current eating and exercise routine then you do not need to follow this book.

If you have heart problems, high cholesterol, diabetes or any other kind of physical problem, are pregnant, or have been forbidden to eat certain foods for medical reasons, please consult your doctor before employing any of the advice in this book.

If your doctor has prescribed you medication that requires you to eat three meals daily then do not skip meals as per this book.

If your doctor has forbidden you from sitting in the sun because of a skin condition, then do not follow the sunbathing passage in this book.

I do not take responsibility for any weight gain, physical injury, or other negative consequences that happen to you after reading this book.

*Great Body No Diet* was written from my personal experience so it does not promise excessive weight loss for obese people. However, if they read the book now, they will gain insights that can help in certain areas and can use the knowledge to maintain their new weight achieved through diet and exercise.

# INTRODUCTION

A great body does not have to be a particular size or shape because we are all different. It does not necessarily have to be thin or look like the body of a Hollywood star; nor does it need to have a six-pack.

Therefore, let us first agree on a mutual definition.

## A Great Body Is:
- Healthy
- Energetic
- Functioning perfectly
- Connected to and controlled by the mind
- Fit
- Flexible
- Coordinated
- Balanced
- Able to control pleasure
- Appealing to a partner
- Soft

## A Great Body Has:
- A robust immune system
- A functional digestive system
- Endurance
- Excellent posture

- Strong lean muscles
- Proportional curves

Once you agree and accept that happiness with your body comes from having these qualities, as opposed to a skinny figure, then kindly carry on reading and aim for a great body!

# The Formula

The formula for success is basic and easy to remember; it must always be kept in mind so you will stay balanced. Refer to it at all times; it is your *mission statement*!

We all love to lose weight, and we all love to save money, right? Well, the formula for losing weight is the opposite of the formula for saving money.

Formula for saving money: *Spend less than you make.*
Formula for losing weight: ***Burn more than you eat.***

To save money, you spend less than your total income and save the rest.

To lose weight, you spend your total income and more.

If you always aim to burn more than you eat, you can sometimes eat more than the average 2,000 to 3,000 calories required daily, as long as you commit to burning it off in the future.

Most diets inform you that in order to lose weight, you need to reduce your daily caloric intake, and they say that your intake should be the same everyday.

However, these diets are not practical because throughout the week, as your level of activity fluctuates, your body needs replenishment accordingly, so on certain days you need to consume more calories, whereas on other days, fewer calories are required.

Let us look at an example:

A woman goes hiking for three hours and burns 1,000 calories; that day, she eats food worth 2,500 calories. The next day, she stays home reading and ends up consuming food worth 1,800 calories. The third day, she makes love to her husband or goes out dancing and burns 400 calories and eats food worth 2,000 calories. Her total intake in three days is 6,300 calories. Assuming that an average woman burns 2,000 calories daily without any sports activity, this means that she has burned 6,000 + 1,400 (from hiking and dancing) = 7,400 calories.

She actually had a nice workout to tone her body, lost an extra 1,100 calories, and got to eat what she likes without restricting herself to a certain amount of calories per day.

I am only referring to calculations of calories so you can understand the concept; with this book you will not be required to count calories.

To stay within the formula, think of what you eat weekly, not on a daily basis, giving yourself more time to burn intake.

If you eat too much skip meals or increase your activity level to burn intake. You will understand this concept better as you continue reading.

Take your time while reading the rest of the book, so that you can gradually absorb the knowledge instead of skimming through and not remembering it well later. The information all ties in together to work for you, so half the knowledge will not be sufficient for success. Besides, you might have been struggling with this challenge your entire life and you survived, so now that you have the answers, relax and enjoy the rest of your life. You really only have two choices: continue as you are and complain or adapt to a new lifestyle and rejoice.

In *Appendix 1* on page 151, you will find cooking methods and recipes to get you started in cooking, followed by *Appendix 2* which has a shopping list that you can always refer to.

In *Appendix 3* on page 163, you will find more information on the research I conducted, and some of the results that were derived.

In *Appendix 4* on page 167, you will find comments, hints and tips that some survey respondents shared while answering the questionnaire.

In *Appendix 5* on page 171, you will find a list of headings of all the passages that you will read in the book, this will help you in future if you want to look up any information that you found useful.

\* \* \*

# 1

# THOUGHTS

Change or Adjust Thoughts about Yourself, Your Body, and Food

The amazing thing is that if you want to have a great body, or nearly anything in life, it all starts in your mind and with your thoughts. That is why this chapter is so long.

We are not trying to trick the mind or the body; on the contrary, because we know our mind so well, we are working with it to get the best results.

## Thoughts about Yourself

### Accept Yourself as You Are
By accepting yourself, you are embracing your uniqueness while making peace with God for creating you as He did. He must have done so for a reason that you will one day understand. (If you have a different belief system, you may think of it whenever I mention God).

## Love Yourself

In loving yourself just as you are, you will find relief and the hostility will vanish. In turn, your energy, determination, and willingness will be focused on what you *can* change.

When you love yourself, the world will love you; when you hate yourself, the world will hate you. The reason this happens is because everything you say and do is in line with how you truly feel about yourself.

Count your blessings every day, and you will start seeing that you have much more than you thought you did.

When you learn to love yourself genuinely, you will rarely harm your body with food, tobacco, or other things; you will treat yourself *right*.

Be happy! Happiness gives you energy to love your life and make something out of it.

## Forgive Yourself

Forgive yourself for treating your body the way you did for all the years that have passed, knowing that it was not very healthy or nice. Forgive yourself for the bad words you said about yourself, your body, your beauty, and promise yourself that from now on you will speak nicely to *you*. This will give you inner peace, and that feeling will spread out to everyone and everything in your life.

## Your Attractiveness Is in Your Soul Energy and Inner Beauty

In general, people are attracted to positive vibes and confidence. It is true that an attractive body can pull attention to itself fast and first, but that is only momentary; soul energy is what keeps the attraction long term. Besides, placing so much importance on external appearance distracts us from the real work we are supposed to be doing on our inner beauty.

Knowing that, focus on how you treat others, be helpful, be nice, and think good thoughts toward them. This is how you create, give, and receive positive energy.

If you are confident and happy with yourself regardless of your weight, enthusiasm will radiate from your center. This draws souls toward you because they feel good in your presence.

Genuine self-confidence does not come from a specific look; it is a result of your achievements. In addition to reaching the big goals you set for yourself, you can do small things that make your soul feel lighter, such as forgiving a friend or relative you lost along the way, developing your personality to become a better person, building long-lasting relationships, and giving.

## Our Differences Make the World Cosmopolitan
If we all looked like Barbie and Ken, life would be boring. People are different, and that is what makes the world so interesting. As Napoleon once said, "*Il faut de tout pour faire un monde*," meaning, *A bit of everything is needed to make up a world*. So that is why there are tall people, short people, blondes, brunettes, and so on.

Not everyone likes thin or voluptuous people, short or tall people, blondes or brunettes. People have different tastes. As long as the one you value likes you as you are, you will be secure and happy.

Admire how many different types of people there are around you when you are waiting for a train or just walking about in a mall.

Embrace your unique look instead of wanting to look like someone else. You should not want to be different than what you are; you should want to be you! You are not perfect from head to toe, no one is, but we all highlight our attractiveness.

If you like being voluptuous, and some people genuinely love it, then enjoy your body as it is.

**Allow Time for the Change to Happen**

There is no time frame for achieving a great body, because we are all different and the amount of time it takes will vary for each person. Most likely, it will require more than just a few months to see major results, but it will surely work. You will need to apply it for your lifetime. Luckily, it is not a diet!

With a long-term goal such as changing your body, work on creating a routine and allow time for the new knowledge and habits to manifest. Change will happen if you really believe in yourself and are determined.

Life is all about change; we see it in weather, trends, rules, and laws. We live it, so why can't we change? I believe that with determination, we can change to what we believe we deserve to be.

If you mess up once in a while, forgive yourself. If you go back to the gym after years of being away from it, give yourself time to reconnect with your muscles. Your brain has a muscle-memory system that allows you to remember its capabilities, that is how we are able ride a bike years after having stopped. If you are trying to rid yourself of old habits, be patient. We are creatures of habit, and we can adopt new ones easily. Mind you, sometimes you actually do like the bad habits, but I will show you how to like the good ones instead.

Some of the things we learned from our parents or others will have to be updated, so do not hang on to old beliefs. Ask God to give you patience again—like you used to have when you were a child, as you might have lost it somewhere along the way. Take your time adapting to your new direction and while losing the kilos you want to lose. That way, your skin will have enough time to adjust to your new shape.

**Be Aware of Your Mood**

Sometimes you find yourself in a bad mood and you direct all the blame toward your weight or how you look; when you do this, you start the negative-thinking process. Do not do that! Ever! You must immediately stop and think, *I will not allow myself to talk to me like that.* Realize that you are in a bad mood, and think of something else. Use positive thoughts to create positive emotions or try to figure out what is really bothering you. Do not take it out on food.

**Stand Up For Yourself**
If any of these people in your life—your spouse, mother, father, guardian, friend, or partner—are interfering with what you eat or telling you what you should and should not eat, you need to stop them nicely because it is none of their business. If people call you names, they are being uncivilized. No matter what they say or do, you are the one who will make the change and it is not up to them. They care about you and do not want to see you develop health problems as you grow older, but they are not helping by constantly interfering. You can see yourself in the mirror and know exactly what is going on. Set boundaries gently for comments that make you feel uncomfortable.

**Ignore Chauvinistic People**
If you are overweight, when you walk into a room and someone gives you dirty looks, you might assume that it is because of how you look, but you cannot read minds, what if that person is having a bad day?

However, there are mean, racist, and superficial people out there, who might actually direct their anger toward you by saying nasty things. Truth is they are the ones with the problem. Do not feel sorry for yourself; instead, feel sorry for them. As difficult as it may be, wish these bullies light and love and forgive them. Then transform their anger into good energy for your soul. Besides, why should you care about what these people think of you? How they see the world is their problem and you will not be able to change them, so just ignore them without letting their comments enter your mind or soul.

**Visit a Poor Country**
When I first met my husband we discussed this book, and he had a funny way of looking at things. He said, "If overweight people were to visit a poor country, their perspective would change and they would probably lose weight." He is concerned about the health of his fellow Americans.

He was athletic in his youth and knows a lot about the body. He works out regularly and does not eat if he is not hungry. He only occasionally eats the things he likes that are less healthy.

On another note he said, "If spoiled or depressed people visit a poor country and see how less fortunate people live, the former would be happier with their own lives."

# Thoughts about Your Body

Appreciate your body, treat it right, love it just the way it is, and be grateful for all that it does for you. It has to last you approximately 80 years or more. So if you are 50 years old now and are reading this book, it means you still have an average of 30 years to enjoy your body and live happily ever after without diets or worries.

**Why Do You Want a Great Body?**
Surely lots of you will have different answers, such as for health, self-confidence, acceptance, or attracting and keeping a partner. The first two answers are good, as for acceptance and keeping a partner, those will not depend on your looks but on how you treat others.

If you want a great body to attract everyone's attention, well, I can tell you that being the center of attention can confuse you, waste your time, or get you off track.

How about this answer? "I want to have a great body to feel confident and comfortable; I want to eat without spoiling my body, fight bacteria and disease, and have enough strength to face life."

## Say No to Weight-Loss Surgeries

If you are considering a weight-loss surgery, it is as though you are trying to resolve the real problem with the click of a button. There is no quick fix operation, pill, or magic tea that can cause your food temptations to vanish. Let us not get into the endless list of complications associated with these methods. The real problem is the eating habits you developed over the years, and it will take some work on your part in order to change your lifestyle. It is not hard work, just consistent work. This book's plan is easy to follow, and the results will last forever.

If you already had an operation, do not regret it; your body will adapt so just move forward and start thinking of a lifestyle change and then begin living it.

## Find Your Ideal Weight

Not every person of a certain height and age must be of the same weight. Some people have thicker bones; others have bigger muscles; some have bigger skulls; and so on. Therefore, fat is not the only thing that is determining your total weight. As you read this book and work on restructuring your body, look at yourself in the mirror every once in a while to see the results. When you lose some weight and it all seems proportional and you are satisfied with your figure, you have reached your ideal weight. Note that number down, and stay on it or go back to it if you ever get off track.

I found that my ideal weight is 58 kilograms (128 pounds) for a 1.70 m height (5 ft. 6 in.). When I lost 2 kilos (4.5 pounds), I had a bony look, and when I gained 2 extra kilos, I felt uncomfortable in my skin and in my clothes.

## Your Body Is the Vehicle of Your Soul

Your body houses your soul and carries it from place to place. What a miracle!

It is the best temple you can ever own. It is all yours and is a reminder that you are right now in life, alive and well. Experiencing the physical world through your senses is your link to the universe; taste and smell are senses that allow you to enjoy flavors. Once you learn how to drive your vehicle, it can take you to the places you want to go and will require plenty of energy to keep up with your demands.

If there is a problem with your body, your soul will not feel at ease, even if you have all the money in the world. A healthy body is the most basic need in your life; attain it.

Love and adore your body. Look at yourself in the mirror while you are in your underwear and admire your body just the way it is. Do not be shy if you are starting to look good. Your beauty is God's gift and creation. It may never be perfect; there might be a bit of cellulite or a few stretch marks, but rarely do people care about detail. No one has it all, so make the best of what you have!

As you look in the mirror, start to figure out which areas need more work and focus on those. Visualize your new shape, and keep it in mind as a goal. Of course, you need to be realistic and know what your body can become. In time, even a year later, slowly but surely, you will achieve it.

Dance around; jump around; feel the freedom from the negative thoughts you had about your body. Only see it in a positive light, and see it improving. Regain your real energy!

## Lose the Weight One Last Time

If you have a lot of weight to lose, over 45 kilos (100 pounds), I suggest that you first read this book and start applying it in a more intense form, meaning, *burn much more than you eat*. If you feel that nothing at all is changing, you may need to use another method or diet that you know will work on you. Lose half your target, and then use this book to lose the remaining weight; after that, you will only need to burn what you eat, instead of worrying about the extra fat you used to have before. So relax; you will never put on that weight again.

**The Belly**
According to the research I conducted, 70 percent of people answered that they do not like their bellies, stomachs, guts, or love handles, and most of them were men.

I have observed that people remember their belly mostly after they finish eating a meal; they start talking about how they want to get rid of it. It is good to want to work on this challenge, but please do not use this time to remember it, because worry and negative thinking after a meal take away its nourishment, and it becomes an uncomfortable presence.

To get rid of your belly, you must understand what is causing you to have it so that you can work through that. Fat is getting stored around your waist because you are eating more than you are burning, so the liver does not have time to catch up. Also, your stomach size has become larger due to past large meals, causing the skin covering it—i.e., your belly—to expand into a larger size, which can also be dealt with, as your elastic-like stomach can shrink to a normal size, once you begin burning more than you eat.

Additionally, the muscles around your waist, front and back, are weak, so they are dropping this part of your body forward. Strengthening these muscles is key, but do not aim for this to happen fast. Please just seek a normal level of strength for now. Begin by mentally connecting with those muscles to reactivate them, so that you can control them with your mind again. Getting rid of your belly must happen slowly so that your muscles will take their time to grow, and your skin will have time to adjust to the new shape.

Whatever the reasons may be, to get rid of your belly, start by holding it in 24 hours a day, seven days a week, while sitting, walking, working, eating, dancing, driving, and *especially* while exercising, or else it will *bulge out*. Holding it in *is* a continuous workout.

I know this sounds crazy or even hard to do at the moment because it is big, but the muscles need to be trained starting now. Do not hold it in too deep, only 50 percent inward, so that you can leave space for your lungs to expand while breathing. It will hurt now, but believe me, in a month or more, it will hurt to let go of it because you will be so used to holding it in. You will see the change in time. In the future, you will have so much control because your mind will reconnect with those muscles and you will feel confident.

The second thing you need to do to decrease your belly size is to shrink the size of your stomach, which was originally about as big as your fist. This can happen gradually, so once your stomach goes back to a normal size, the fat around your belly will be used up as extra energy for the body and melt away. Here is how to shrink the size of your stomach naturally:

- Start shrinking the size of your meals to a reasonable average size. Suppose you eat two main courses in one meal; make that one main course plus four to five more medium bites. The less you overstretch your stomach by overeating, the more it starts to shrink.

- Avoid drinking anything at all while eating meals, and do not drink anything after your meals, for at least 45 minutes to an hour after food, or until you feel the meal has diminished in your stomach. Always drink water *before* you eat food or sweets, and if there is something else you feel like drinking, especially beer, have it before the food or one hour afterwards.

- Strengthen your back muscles because they too can help bring back a normal shape. You can do this with swimming, back-ups, or any other type of exercise that suits your shape.

- Take long walks while holding your belly in. Breathe deep and walk slowly. Be sure that you are connecting with your belly muscles. This may be easier than trying to do sit-ups. No matter what the weather outside is like, walk; this is the best thing you can do for yourself. Make walking a long-term habit, take a friend, do not come back and check yourself out in the mirror in the hope of having lost weight after one walk, be realistic.

- There are exercises to make your waist smaller and some sit-ups and stretches to strengthen your abdominal muscles. Search for stomach stretching and exercises on the Internet, and there are some examples in *Chapter 5* of this book.

- Read the next section: "Waste or Waist?"

- Lie down on your back, and hug your belly. It is part of you; do not hate it; do not separate yourself from it. Massage your belly gently giving positive energy toward your gut and visualize yourself melting and releasing all the fat that was stored in it. Visualize your belly shrinking to the size you want and your intestines and skin adjusting to the new shape, while your muscles take control, and carry you better in the future. Most important, *truly* believe that you will conquer it.

- Finally, the moment you think, *My tummy is big*, and you begin to get into a rut about it, hold it in!

## Waste or Waist?

A very good way to save yourself from overeating, when there is hesitation, is to ask yourself: "Waste or waist?" meaning, "Do I dump the extra food into myself and increase my 'waist' size, or do I dump the food in the 'waste' bin?" The second option is always best because you are not a waste bin. I know your mother taught you to finish your plate when you were a kid even though you felt full; that was important for you then as you needed to develop your brain and body, but you will have to let go of this habit now because you are fully grown. It is important for you to know that taking in anything extra will expand your stomach, and may turn into fat. If you are already full, have a few more bites and throw the rest away or store it in the fridge for the next meal.

For example, if you really feel like a gourmet burger for lunch, drink lots of water before you have it and then cut it into two pieces. If half the burger fills you up, then stop right there and think; *Waste or waist?* You can have another quarter of it, give the other half to someone at the table, or take a doggy bag home. If you ate the entire burger, skip dinner, because you will not feel hungry anyhow. Perhaps, you could have a fruit salad or anything you think is right or maybe nothing at all; you are smart enough to figure out what is best according to your situation that day.

## Let the Fat Go

If you already have excess fat, you are probably holding onto it in your mind as well; do what is necessary and release it mentally and physically. There will always be food for you to eat. Do not think that any meal you are having is the last meal you will ever eat. Let the food go into your mouth and out of your body without storing any of it.

## Heat Melts Grease

Have you noticed how difficult it is to wash dishes with cold water? On the other hand, *hot* water melts grease easily and quickly. The grease inside our food and body requires a hot temperature to dissolve it, which is why you must exercise. Exercising generates heat inside your body to burn fat.

# Thoughts that Are Informative

### Create Your Own Physical Activity Routine
The fact is that most of us gain weight as we grow older. The main reason is because we decrease the amount of physical activity and become accustomed to using our brains more and our bodies less. In high school, we were forced to attend physical education classes, but after graduation, some of us did not maintain this discipline.

### Advertising Is Targeting You
Advertising, especially in the United States, is so powerful and beautiful to watch. The ads are so smart and creative, they can completely hypnotize people. There are hundreds of food companies advertising their products so they can make a lot of money out of their target audience: *you*! You are bombarded with these ads, and they usually work by creating a craving in you. Once you know this, you will not be fooled anymore and can resist any ad. Be strong!

Advertising can be useful when you allow it to give you creative ideas on what to eat, what products are doing well in the market, and what is new.

### Diets Are Short-Term, Not Lifetime Solutions
Some dieticians can give you a diet now that will make you lose 10 kilos (22 pounds) in one month. Suppose it takes you two months to reach your target; then what will you do afterward? Go back to your old eating habits? You cannot remain on a diet your entire life. Think of the lifestyle I am advocating as a long-term plan.

Gaining and losing weight repeatedly, too quickly like in liposuction, or unnaturally will spoil your skin and that may call for another operation.

Release fat slowly and healthily; that is the ideal way, because it allows time for the skin to regenerate as much as possible. Our bodies have an amazing self-healing ability and can make tremendous progress if given ample time to do so.

Do not hold negative images in your mind of how your skin will look, you will cross that bridge once you get to it.

With diets, you lose your physical energy and cannot cope with daily life. All you do is think about food. With this book, you will forget about food; it will always be the last thing on your mind because you will have solved its mystery.

One of the reasons diets do not work is because they are not realistic. They tell you to weigh and measure everything. How can you do that while you are traveling or at big events? In addition, the moment you are told not to eat certain things, you start feeling frustrated as if your freedom has been taken away. We are constantly told to be in control of ourselves in other areas of our lives; food may be the only space and time where we are truly free, so nobody wants to give that up. When you want to eat, think of something nice that you like and enjoy this pleasure. A famous singer once went on a popcorn diet; that was all she ate for many days. She lost several kilograms, but imagine how many vitamins and nutrients her body was missing after that. She is a very energetic person, so no worries for her, but if you try something like that, who knows? You might faint.

Another woman I know went on a sleeping diet; this means she slept at least 16 hours a day to reduce her appetite, because upon waking, one does not have a big appetite. It worked on her, but imagine how depressing that must have been!

There was another diet that was popular for a while, and it involved a strict menu during the week and a day off on the weekend. The dieters would feel the frustration all week long and then binge the entire day on their day off of the diet.

We are thankful and grateful to doctors, nutritionists, and dieticians for all the research they have done over the years on food and how many calories exist in certain foods. Without that knowledge, we would have no clue at all what happens in our system, but let us face it; no one has yet come up with a realistic and long-term solution that works with human nature. Let us look at the big picture and stop going into details about the chemistry behind everything.

*Survey Responses about Dieting and Types of Diets*

- 80% of people do not like diets.

- 53% of people stated that diets made them stressed and put constraints on them and they relapsed later or that they did not believe in them because they did not work.

- 22% do not like diets because they like food and do not like to deprive themselves of indulgences.

- 20% of people like diets because they keep them healthy, balanced, and purified.

*Post-diet Results*

- 80% of people lost weight while dieting.

- 46% said they gained the weight back, and the remaining 54% did not. This shows that in some cases diets do have a long-term effect.

- Some people lost amazing amounts of weight; two men lost 60 kilograms (132 pounds) once and for all, and a woman in her early thirties lost 45 kilograms (99 pounds) twice in her life but could not keep the weight off.

## Gained or Lost Weight Shows after a Few Weeks

When you are on the path of losing weight, it will take time to show on your body, sometimes two weeks or more. The reverse is also true; if you ate a lot for a few days, it will not immediately show on your body and you have time to burn it off before it settles, what a blessing!

## Working Out Makes You Heavier at First

As soon as you start working out after not having done so for a while, your muscles, which were asleep and flat, will begin puffing up and getting bigger and heavier. This will make your total weight heavier, and you will appear wider when you look in the mirror. Since you do not realize that this only happens at the beginning of your new lifestyle, you might get discouraged and stop your workout and diet routine entirely, thinking that nothing is really happening and that there is no hope for you. No! Keep going! This *is* the right track, the only track, and you are on it! Once your muscles get bigger, they will help you burn the fat on top of them. They will carry your body and speed up your metabolism. With time, your body will look amazing and be thinner. It is only a matter of time before you get to where you want to go!

## Do Not Deny Yourself Completely; Indulge Occasionally

When you go to dieticians, they do tests on you and start making a list of the things you are not allowed to eat. This is why you went to see them in the first place, and the reason they have a job. Some honest or advanced dieticians actually advise you not to stop eating any type of food, because you need carbohydrates, fats, and proteins for your brain function, muscle activity, skin, hair, eye, and liver vitality.

Keep this healthy intake at 70 percent, and the remaining 30 percent for indulgence.

## Hard Work Requires Energy

If you are working really hard, you will need a lot of energy to be able to cope and continue, especially if you are sleeping fewer hours than usual; this means you will need a bit more food because of those extra hours of being awake and working. If you are on a diet while being pressured at work, you will lose energy and will not feel happy. The purpose of this book is to keep your energy high, but not your weight. You need to feel strong, so eat a bit from each food group, such as carbohydrates, proteins, and fat, and make sure you are drinking enough water.

I had a realization recently involving energy; it is that your energy really comes from you and not the food you eat. Your energy comes from your dedication and commitment to being alive, so you could be eating really healthily but have no energy toward life, and the opposite is also true; you could be eating unhealthily but have so much energy for life and what you are doing. The problem is that in the long run, eating unhealthily and working really hard may burn you out, so you are better off being dedicated to life and to eating healthy.

## Your Body Knows What It Needs

Ask your body what it needs to eat, not what it wants to eat, and it will most likely want something healthy. For it to be healthy, it requires certain elements. Your mind knows what is needed and when, depending on the state of your system, so it will trigger a desire for it.

Open your fridge and ask your body what it needs, and you will be surprised that you will find yourself looking at the answer; sometimes an image can pop into your mind and you will find that you do not have it at home. You can always buy it the same day or the next day at the store. For example, if you feel a craving for cucumbers or watermelon, this could signify dehydration that might lead to constipation if not treated in time.

Before going food shopping, while writing your list, ask your body what it needs. Suddenly, you might find yourself writing: spinach, eggs, and apples. Those are the things your mind is telling you to buy for your body, and you will surely enjoy eating them knowing this.

Keala Carter, an American holistic nutritionist and personal trainer, shared her thoughts on what she thinks is the main problem in her country. She said that people do not listen to themselves or their bodies; they have lost the connection between mind and body, and have become accustomed to listening to others instead.

If you want to reconnect your mind with your body, I would suggest meditation and yoga to strengthen your breathing and quiet your stress; that way, you can hear your inner voice more clearly. There are special workshops to get you started, such as The Art of Living, designed by the Guru Purnima H. H. Sri Sri Ravi Shankarji[1].

I once attended this workshop in Dubai. It lasted a week and we learned breathing techniques, exercises, yoga, and ways to mentally deal with the stresses of life. They taught us to eat our fruits before lunch so that they go down quicker and line the stomach to help digestion. We were asked to be vegetarian and to stop consuming alcohol, coffee, tea and smoking cigarettes for the week while we were in training. I recommend this course if you ever want a life change.

**Channels of Melted Fat**

After fat melts, it leaves the body through sweat and in the urine; so sometimes over urinating could be a sign of weight loss as a result of burning lots of energy. (Be careful because over urinating could also be a sign of a bladder infection. Go see a doctor if you feel pain in that area of your body.)

---

1 http://www.artofliving.org/us-en

Avoid deodorants that block the pores under your armpits resulting in no excretion of sweat because this is unnatural to the process of releasing fat.

Scrub your body during each shower to get rid of dead skin and keep pores open for sweat to pass easily. Avoid the body sponges that create bacteria, the plastic ones are best. After the shower, apply cream on your skin to keep it hydrated and soft.

**You Do Not Require the Same Food Quantity Everyday**
This is a positive thought, because it means that during the days when you eat less, you will be burning what you ate over the few days or weeks that passed. Let us look at a few situations:

- Your appetite for hot food decreases during summer. *Note: in hot weather, increase your intake of fruits and water to remain hydrated and energized.*

- In winter, your body feels cold and requires heat; that heat can be created from the energy in food, and that is why your appetite grows during this season. Remain active and you will not store fat from the increase in food intake.

- Before a woman's menstrual cycle, her body retains water and she appears fatter than usual, she feels like eating a lot, and when she gets her period, her desire to eat decreases (this is true in many women but not all). Her body is going through a big change so it is perfectly okay to overeat during those days.

- If you are in love, you tend to eat less because of the excitement you are feeling. If you just ended a relationship, you may overeat or not eat at all; each person is different.

- During the Christmas season or other yearly celebrations, you attend parties where lots of good, sometimes homemade food is served, or you may go to a large buffet at a restaurant. Those days you eat more, but do not worry; if you follow the tips in this book, you will go through all these occasions smoothly and be in control of your weight.

- Some people eat less when they are busy; this is to avoid feeling heavy and tired. Keep drinking water on busy days, and make sure you handle your hunger well at the end of your day so that you do not overeat or eat the wrong things.

- When you go back to exercising, during the first few weeks, you will feel hungrier than usual and might eat more. After a short while, you will be able to readjust to normal-sized meals.

- Some people eat more on weekends and less during the week and vice versa.

Depending on your activities, follow your logic and instinct when it comes to eating and use the formula to balance.

**Food for the Body Is Like Fuel for the Car**
Whenever you drive your car, do you stop every few miles and refill the tank?

Most of you wait until it is nearly empty before filling it up again; it is the same with your stomach. Wait until you have consumed the energy from the food you have eaten before eating your next meal.

**If You Abuse Your Freedom, You Lose Yourself**
Let us face it; this book gives you freedom. Remember not to abuse your freedom because that is how you lose

yourself. Remain in control and balanced; and be honest with yourself.

## Consume Fizzy Drinks Rarely
If you place a tooth in fizzy Cola, it melts after four days. That is why people are subconsciously addicted to fizzy drinks; it helps them to digest the food they eat. The downside to fizzy drinks is the amount of sugar they contain; they also cancel out the vitamins and minerals in a meal, so your body will not get all the benefits. Therefore, drink them rarely.

# Thoughts to Move You in the Right Direction

There will be a day when you decide to go healthy, and from that point on, when faced with choices, you will tend to gravitate toward the healthier option.

## Change Your Motto from Lazy to Active
Laziness is the most destructive human trait; it is your worst enemy. You must do all that is within your power to get rid of it. The good news is that laziness is more of a *thought* than a physical problem. You must be able to fight off lazy thoughts by immediately remembering that you are active. Make it so that anytime there is a beneficial activity and your mind tries to sway you from it, identify the thought and eliminate it.

> *Tip: Anything that needs to be done, do it with a smile! Do it with energy!* ☺

## Live Spontaneously
When you follow a diet, it tells you exactly what to eat and when. Where is the excitement in that? I like to live

spontaneously; I like to ask my body what it needs and my tongue what it feels like. I might be in a restaurant where they have a special way of cooking a dish—for example, paella—so I order that. Do not be afraid of trying new things; yes, some days, you might end up ordering something that you dislike, but you also might discover something very tasty that you never knew existed.

## Encourage Yourself without Creating Pressure

You may be putting pressure on yourself; everybody does it. You may be telling yourself things like "I *have to* lose weight; I *should* exercise." The words *have* to and *should* make things seem like a *must* instead of a *want* to do. Instead, think: I *want* to be healthy; I *want* to exercise.

## Give Thanks Before and After You Eat

Before you eat a meal, say Grace. When you finish eating, be thankful to God, to the chef, and to yourself, instead of moaning about how much fat, carbohydrates or calories it contains. Believe me, one meal cannot possibly change your form. On the contrary, it will be beneficial to you when you are thanking the universe for giving you this food for your survival. Ask God to bless you with energy from this food that will help you stay strong so you can face life.

## Your Logic Will Guide You

Eat according to your logic and intuition. No one is with you 24 hours a day watching what you are eating, especially not your nutritionist, so be your own nutritionist and use your intelligence and common sense. While deciding what to eat, be truthful with your answers.

We are all incredible beings with superb logic and intelligence. We feel good when we are using our brains to survive and be happy.

The reason this book makes so much sense and may sound familiar to you is because it is addressing your logic.

## Ask God to Help You

While praying, always thank God for the graceful body He gave you. Ask Him to bless your system and for it to work in perfect coordination until the last day.

God will surely help you; He is always there for us. God made our bodies, and they were made for eating. Temptation exists for us to strengthen our will power.

## Figure Out what Needs Work

You may be making a series of mistakes, like eating late, not breathing well, eating oily food, or not exercising. Or maybe you gained weight a long time ago and never got rid of it. Whatever your story, try to figure out logically what you are not doing right as you read this book. Figure out why you are not losing the weight you want to lose, and start working on solving the problem, but give yourself time. It is not magic.

If you need help, you can always visit my website www. greatbodynodiet.com and contact me. I am working on offering group workshops and one-on-one coaching to guide people.

## Skipping Meals Is Okay

You were taught:

1.  To never skip meals—i.e., eat three times a day even if you are not hungry.

2.  To never skip the same meal, such as breakfast, lunch, or dinner, on a daily basis.

I totally agree with the second part of this statement but not the first. Skipping the same meal everyday does not work with this book because sometimes you need that meal to replenish your system. The main reason you were told not to skip meals at all is because your metabolism slows down, and your body will hold onto everything you eat in your next meal because it was starved earlier. I am against this thinking and this habit of eating thrice a day even when not hungry, and if you disagree with me; this book may not work for you at all.

The main reason is logical; this statement is assuming that you are eating three reasonable sized meals daily, but let us face it, we sometimes eat more than the reasonable amount, so if you eat three large meals a day when you are not hungry and when your body is not asking for it, there is only one thing that can happen to you: you will gain weight. Less intake means less weight, so you are better off eating two large meals instead of three.

Also, when do you expect your liver to break down the extra fat that is sitting on your waist or in other parts of your body? Your liver is always so busy digesting the three meals and snacks that you are constantly eating every day, that it almost never has time to deal with the extra fat in your body.

I have tried and tested this over and over again and have always come to the same conclusion; skipping meals is okay when there is sufficient food in your system. Here is one example:

You eat a huge or heavy meal, which sometimes happens at events like weddings or Christmas parties. This means that it will take you more time than the usual four to five hours to digest. You will know when this happens, because when it is time to eat your next meal, whether breakfast, lunch, or dinner, you will not feel hungry at all. *That* is the moment you should decide to skip a meal. Even after digestion, you must wait to get hungry or wait for some time to use up the energy from the food before you have your next meal, i.e., *burn before you eat*. Be sure to drink lots of water for digestion in these cases. This will become a habit later as you get used to this lifestyle.

Follow your logic and ask yourself if you are hungry; do not just follow the clock and eat because it happens to be lunchtime. It may not be *your* lunchtime. This is the time when burning takes place and you are able to stay within the formula: *burn more than you eat*.

*Note: Do not skip a meal if your last few meals were light. Eat healthy meals daily so that you always have energy and will not feel faint.*

**No Scale at Home**
Do not keep a scale in your home unless it is used solely to weight luggage. If you weight your body, you will obsess about the details. Muscles weigh more than fat, so you may not weigh less in kilos but your body may look so much better. Looking at the scale keeps you focused on your weight. But having a great body is not about the kilos; it is about how toned, agile, fit, strong, and coordinated you are.

**Think Clockwise**
Just like time, everything we do is clockwise, and food is what keeps us moving, fuelling our system for survival. So if you occasionally overeat, remember that time does not stop; there is still a chance in the future to burn off the energy. We are creatures constantly consuming and expending energy while talking, walking, driving, listening, reading, working, and sitting, as time is passing clockwise, our blood is flowing through our veins, and energy is required and used up. Brain activities burn like

exercise does, so remain focused while you are doing brainwork, especially while studying or working on solving a problem.

## Think Confidence, Life, and Breath of Life

Life is made up of moments. In most of your moments smile genuinely, breathe deep, and think to yourself, *I love life and I am happy*. Be thankful because you have access to good food, this is a privilege that not everybody has.

You see the world with your eyes, and the world sees you through your eyes. They reveal how you feel inside.

## Breathing Is Like Fuel for Burning Food

Just like air that contains oxygen keeps a fire burning, air keeps your metabolism running and burning energy in your body. You must use your full lung capacity to make the best of your body; if you use half your lungs, you are not connecting to your entire body. So we can safely say that breathing *fresh* air properly helps in weight loss.

Do you ever wonder why you do not taste food when you have a cold? It is because you do not smell it; by breathing, you get to smell it and therefore taste it properly. Breathing while eating does help you enjoy food. Mind you, your nose tubes must be open and clean to taste food even better.

As far as I can remember, my father would always walk into a room, slide the window slightly open, and say, "How can you guys breathe in here?" He used to tell me to open the window before sleeping. It was amazing because the nights I would forget to do that, I would wake up with a headache, feeling tired and not wanting to get up.

Open the windows in your home to get fresh air. Do not breathe the same air all day long, especially in winter when the heater is on. If you keep breathing the same air, it can make you lazy and tired. If you cannot open a window, then go outside for fresh air every hour or turn on the air-conditioning if you live somewhere hot.

Some of today's cooking stoves that use gas have a pilot that stays on all the time; it is like having candles constantly lit in your kitchen, burning all the oxygen and omitting gas in your living space. If you have one of those stoves, please do not keep the pilots on all day, light them when you want to cook.

Happiness and breathing are linked. If you are unhappy or sad, you tend to breathe slower while arching your body forward and blocking your air passage; this slow breathing will only leave you feeling worse, as you will add tiredness to your problem. Straighten up your posture while breathing, and try to get out of your mood. Sulking is the worst thing you can do to yourself. Go out there and talk about it.

# Thoughts for Success

### Be Reserved about Your New Venture
Do not talk incessantly about what you are doing to change your shape; keep it to yourself. The point is not to think of food anymore; it will be in the back of your mind. It has all been worked out since you are reading and understanding this book, so there is no need to discuss it over again with people. The less you talk about food, the less you think about it.

### Be Ready to Answer Questions
When people ask you what you have done to lose weight, be brief yet nice and answer with a smile, "I am changing my lifestyle when it comes to eating." They may continue, "So are you on a diet?" Answer, "No, I eat a bit of everything." It is no one's business what you eat or do not eat, so why focus on this topic?

There is no need to get into a huge debate and conversation about which school of thought to follow. Each person is entitled to his or her own opinion. Be confident about what you are doing.

If asked whether you work out, say, "Yes I work out twice a week or when I have time."

If they are really curious and want to know what you are doing to change your body, give them a copy of the book, or tell them about it.

**The Frog Story**
(This is a motivational story used in training employees; the author is unknown.)

> There once was a frog race. The frogs were asked to climb up a tower; the first one who reached the top would be the winning frog. They all rushed toward the tower at the sound of a whistle and started climbing upward. Some of them fell down, but others kept going. The ones who fell began shouting, "You will never make it! It's too steep!" More fell down, and others kept climbing. Those who fell began screaming, "It's too high! You will never make it!" And so the rest fell down until there was only one frog left, climbing with difficulty yet still going. The rest of the frogs kept shouting to him, "You will fall like the rest of us did!" Funnily enough, the frog made it and became the winning frog. When the winning frog came back down, the rest were very curious and asked, "How did you win this race?" It turns out this frog was deaf!

Remember this story and remind yourself to be deaf to negative comments from yourself or other people; stay positive and you will succeed ☺.

**Your Job Is Not an Excuse**
You might be giving yourself an excuse for being the way you are, so try to notice if you are using your job or

your working hours as an excuse not to exercise or lose weight.

For example, if you work at a consulting firm, you might be finishing work at midnight each day; this will not allow you time to go to the gym after work. Your best solutions are either to work out in the morning before work or twice on the weekend.

If you do not have a weekend at all because of your workload, be careful because you might be overworking yourself, and this is counterproductive.

## Be a Self-Starter

The most important quality employers look for when hiring new employees is that of being a self-starter. Self-starters are people who make their own schedules on a daily basis and achieve them instead of waiting for someone to tell them what to do. Become a self-starter in every aspect of your life. This will help you achieve all your goals.

## You Are What You Think

You are what you think, and you are what you eat. So if you are eating bad and thinking bad, you will look it! But do not worry, even if you have been doing this your entire life, you can stop right now by simply deciding to drop this habit, just like you would drop a hot piece of coal in your hand, and from now on, continue thinking positive to create good emotions.

Food is a joyful experience, be grateful each time you eat. Once you replace the old thoughts with these new good ones, food will always serve you and will sit nicely in your body like the wonderful thoughts in your mind.

If you *think* slim, you will *be* slim. While speaking, you might be constantly referring to yourself as fat. How will you ever change your body if this is your state of mind? You are making it seem like it is a permanent thing, but it is not.

Always think to yourself, *I am slim*, even if it is not true yet. Keep thinking it until it manifests in your life.

If someone tells you that you seem to have gained weight, ignore it; do not believe any comment that is not aligned with how you see the new you.

Perhaps you might wake up with a puffy face on some days. It may seem that you have put on weight, but it is most likely not the case; it may just be one of those days or perhaps you have your period and your entire body is puffy or you are retaining water because of humid weather. Even if you know you have gained a little and people notice, laugh about it and say, "Oh yeah, I might have, but it will melt away again; it is temporary."

Be careful which words you are using—for example, "I am starving!" Overall, you are not a starving person; so do not use those heavy words because it might become your excuse for overeating at mealtime. Just say to yourself or others, "I feel like eating something."

## Visualization

It is a very powerful tool that a human being can use to achieve dreams and goals. Learn to use this tool, as it is the key to realizing your goal of a great body. It has been scientifically proven that winning competitions is linked with visualization of winning. Thoughts are vital for your success.

You are what you project of your future. Look at your body in a very positive way. Even if it is not true at the moment or at the beginning of your decision to change, pretend like it is and believe that it will be.

Visualize and dream of the new you; see yourself as being the size you want to be; and think it over and over again. Always keep a vision of how you want to look in your mind, and you will eventually become that vision.

Remember that your charm is in your eyes and in your smile. Smile with your soul, too. One of the survey participants offered a valuable piece of advice: "Smile, and they all smile with you; frown, and no one remains with you."

## Time Is Short

You are lucky that nowadays there is so much you can do, but that is also what makes time feel like it is passing by really fast. In the olden days, there was not much to do but sit and eat, and a meal took at least two hours to complete. Nowadays lunch breaks at work are shorter, so use that to your advantage by eating less, and by encouraging yourself to pack a healthy lunch from home.

## Eating while in a Temporary Bad Mood

If you are upset and eating while thinking of why you are sad, angry, jealous, or whatever negative emotion you may be experiencing, you should stop eating, finish thinking, and then eat, or stop thinking negatively and continue eating. Negative thinking is so heavy that it takes all your energy; goes down like poison in your system; and you will not focus on the taste of the food. You will not feel full and will want to eat more. So have pure thoughts related only to the good taste of the food.

## Eating Must Not Be Followed by Feelings of Guilt

Many people curse themselves after eating something that they really enjoy, whether it is chocolate or a croissant. People feel that way about eating something that is perceived as fattening, when in reality, it is only fattening if abused. And each bite is followed by self-criticism. Why? Stop doing that and respect your being.

Many chocolate advertisements associate *pleasure* with *guilt*, and this messes up the entire experience. The truth is they are associating a horrible feeling, which is guilt, with the beautiful sensation we get from eating chocolate, which is pleasure; these two must not be mixed. We should be thankful and grateful for pleasure.

## Eliminate Negative Thoughts

Negative thoughts are a barrier to success; do not listen to negative affirmations from your past. For example, thoughts like, *My metabolism is slow*, can really affect your positivity toward using up the energy in meals and keeping your body balanced. Whoever told you that? Even if doctors or nutritionists said it, please do not believe that it is permanent. A doctor once told me that my metabolism was slow, and I have proven otherwise.

The traditional way to measure resting metabolic rate (RMR) is to use a standardized formula that factors in your sex, weight, height, and age. One of those formulas is known as the Harris-Benedict equation.

"Many equations just provide rough and dirty ballpark estimates," says Cedric Bryant, Chief Exercise Physiologist for the American Council on Exercise in San Diego.[2]

RMR is the total number of calories your body burns in a day while at rest, carrying out typical body functions, like breathing and pumping blood (involuntary muscle activities). So this means that if you breathe deeper and start exercising, you can increase your RMR. Exercising helps to coordinate the body muscles, both voluntary and involuntary.

Also, we are emotional beings, so for example, getting angry one day can use up a lot of energy (please do not use anger as a weight-loss activity). Finally, look for articles on the Internet on how to speed up your metabolism naturally, you will find plenty of useful information.

Making excuses with thoughts like, *I can't run because of my knee operation.* There are many other ways to exercise. In the meantime, think of an activity that does

---

2 www.newleaffitness.com

not put pressure on your knees, or simply walk fast, swim, or do yoga while omitting some painful postures. Perhaps your knee problem was years ago, and today is a new day. Think, *Mind over matter*, and heal yourself.

Thoughts like, *If I quit cigarettes, I will gain weight.* No! On the contrary, you will have more energy to move and exercise, because you will have more oxygen entering your lungs, so your body will burn food faster. It is a misconception that by stopping cigarettes you will gain kilos. I used to smoke, and I have quit and restarted several times. Each time I quit, I would become so much more active and go hiking, swimming, traveling, and moving at any occasion instead of sitting on the couch and smoking.

*Note: this book will work on smokers and nonsmokers.*

Thoughts like, *No matter what I do, I will always be fat,* are extremely negative, and your chances of success with such thinking are very low. You really have to believe in yourself, your power, intelligence, and your ability to transform your body. This is one of the things in life that you *can* change. Fat melts like butter on a stove once you create the right temperature for it to do so, and your starting point is the normal temperature of the body: 37°C (98.6°F).

After you eat do not think, *This will take so long to digest*; instead, think, *I have eaten food to last me many hours. It is energy to keep me warm and alive and will help me to face my life and challenges.* So thank God and breathe deeply.

Other thoughts to be avoided are these:

- *I will never lose weight*—You have never read this book before, so give it a chance.

- *I am too old to lose weight*—There is no age limit for melting fat.

- *I can never get rid of this fat*—At the right temperature, fat melts and leaves the body.

- *I do not have time to cook at home so I eat out*—Make time to cook; it is much healthier because you know what is going into the meal. Cook at night for the next day, or freeze meals for later. Each step while cooking a meal takes just a few seconds, and while the dish is heating up, you can clean the kitchen.

- *It's hereditary*—Extra weight does not come through your DNA, it is from what you ate in the past.

- *I cannot stand exercising*—Believe me, the feeling on your way out of the gym after a workout is amazing, so when you are doing it right, you will *love* it.

- *I cannot afford a gym membership*—Okay, so go to a public place, like a park or the beach and exercise there, or hike a trail. Working out is nicer outdoors where there is an abundance of fresh air.

- *I do not have time to exercise*—Make time. Besides, it is only going to be twice a week. You can always find one day on the weekend and one day during the week, or two days during the week. The ironic thing is that working out makes you faster at everything you do in your life, so working out will help you create more free time.

- *I am so lazy*—Energy brings on energy, and laziness brings on laziness. This could be the reason you think of yourself this way and are unable to move away from this state of mind, so switch back to energetic mode.

Also, laziness is a thought in your mind; replace it with, *Sometimes I can be lazy if I am very tired; other times, I am full of energy.* When you think lazy thoughts replace them with, *I can do this!*

- *I do not know how to cook, or Men do not cook*—Learn! It is a form of art and science, and no one can please your palette better than you can.

- *I am not supposed to skip meals*—I explained why this is not true earlier.

These negative thoughts need to be plucked out of your mind and replaced with positive affirmations. Just say the opposite of each thought and start believing it, because it is true.

If you have any negative thoughts in your mind that I have not mentioned, please try to notice them, figure out why you have them, from whom you got them, and replace them with positive thoughts forever. Change your thoughts and your life will change.

### Create Good Thoughts
Constantly think positive, *I am an active human being. I am productive. I am wonderful. I am beautiful. I embrace change. I can change.*

The main thoughts you need to have clearly in your mind are about your ability to lose weight and to be thin forever, because it is very possible.

If you get negative thoughts again at any time after you have thrown them away, close your eyes and think positive, *I am a divine being. I control my body with my mind, and I control my thoughts. My body is the instrument of my mind, and it works for me. I can achieve anything I set my mind to. My body is God's creation and a miracle. I am made up of energy. Energy is heat, and that can be used at any time to burn food. I am fast at shopping and have plenty of time to cook. I can always find time to exercise, and if I have physical pain, I can swim or find another means of using my muscles. I can quit smoking and substitute it with a healthy activity.*

## Commitment

Commitment is a very important human pledge, and it requires honesty and trust for it to work.

If you commit to eating something, then commit to burning it off.

Committing to burning fast food is not easy; the fat is so condensed that the body stores it because it cannot break it down. Why do we think that our stomach can break down all the heavy stuff? It is simply illogical. On the other hand, if you happen to eat junk food very rarely, then keep thinking that your body will not hold on to it.

## Embrace the Feeling of Hunger

I came to the conclusion that people do not like the feeling of hunger. It irritates them because they allow it to take over the moment, and as a result, they lose energy and feel cranky. They cannot think of anything except eating. Your thoughts are like wild horses if you do not tame them by controlling them.

Embrace the feeling of hunger when you need to and have no other choice. It is a nice feeling, as it brings you back to your basic need in life, and if you feel hungry, immediately remember many people spend their lives hungry, and thank God that you do not.

Some people are always feeling hungry. This might be because they fill their stomachs to the max, get dehydrated, and the minute the food starts to disappear, the rumbling starts again, so they think they are hungry and keep their stomachs quiet by eating when they do not need to, instead of drinking water. When your stomach makes hunger noises, it is shrinking because it is empty, and that is a good thing; it does not mean you are going to die. Do not let this feeling bother you; on the contrary, be happy.

When you feel hunger and brush it away, you can last for a long time before eating again. Think about those who fast for an entire month every year; they spend all day, an average of 9 hours, working without food or drink, some of them exercise and cook before eating at sunset. They have transformed hunger into something divine and actually are not bothered by it as you might imagine. They are building inner strength by practicing self-restraint. Do you think you can last a couple of hours hungry?

Your mind does its duty and triggers hunger and that is how you know that your system is running on reserves; it is up to you to act on that or not. Of course, you are going to eat sooner or later, so it would be better if you can delay the sooner to later. Right now you are so busy, too busy to eat, so finish what you are doing, and enjoy your meal later. However, do not starve yourself, as you might get dizzy or end up eating too fast at the next meal; you must know your limits.

When you eat in extreme hunger or after sports, the food gets digested quickly. For example, you spent all day waterskiing burning plenty, and have not had anything yet; you left it until nighttime to eat, that is okay, you will digest quicker than usual.

A sure way to delay the hunger feeling is by eating food or snacks that contain fiber. Find out what those are by researching on the Internet and fill your desk drawers at work with high-fiber snacks so that you can last longer.

### Waiting for Pleasures Makes Them More Enjoyable
I am sure that by now you know that food tastes so much better when you are hungry. This basic concept applies to most other things in life; it feels so much better to

sleep when you are very tired, make love when you have waited for it, drink water when you are thirsty (though there are times you must drink even if you are not feeling thirsty), get a massage once a month instead of weekly, or have an alcoholic beverage occasionally so that it gives you a buzz.

Pleasure is a very tricky thing, and caution must be taken so that it never becomes harmful. Enjoy things, but know when to stop and do not allow yourself to be controlled by a pleasure because it may turn into a nasty habit and can then turn into an addiction. Longing for something makes it more pleasurable. Moderation is the best answer here.

## Do Not Cross the Red Line
Your stomach is as big as your fist and can expand when full; Though your stomach size can expand a lot, your red line should be the point where you feel pain from overeating. Never eat until you reach that point. The main reason is because after any meal you should avoid sleep and have energy to do small physical things to kick start digestion, such as playing chess, walking, dishes, etc. If you overate, you are temporarily unable or not wanting to do anything at all, and this slows down your entire cycle, and you will have to wait longer before eating your next meal.

## Knowing and Applying
If you already know something is good for you, why are you not applying it? You are knowingly working against what is right for you. You need to self-construct and not the opposite. Motivate yourself to do what you know is right.

You tell your body what to do, not the opposite. Take yourself seriously. Respect your own authority; you are the boss of you, so listen to and obey the good commands.

Before you approach food, make a conscious decision that you will not be driven by hunger, you will eat at a moderate pace, you will get full, and be satisfied.

**Simply *Be* Healthy**
When your overall state of being is healthy, this means that every thought and action takes you in that direction. Decide that at your core you want to be healthy; things will just fall into place, and the ride will be smoother for you.

# Thoughts about Food

**Use Logic and Experience**
People have different opinions about the same things. For example, I might tell you that drinking water before food is very good for you. One day later you might meet someone and share this thought, and he or she will tell you otherwise. I would say try the things that make sense, and adopt what works for you. This way, you are the one who is deciding.

Also, beliefs about certain things change. For example, one day, science tells us that coffee is very bad for the health, but then a few years down the line, new research proves that coffee is good for us. It becomes confusing. Therefore, rely on your own judgment based on logic and experience. If you notice that consuming a certain food or drink gives you heart palpitations, indigestion, bloating, or any kind of discomfort, then stop consuming it. Basically, become your own scientist and study your body by the process of observation because we are different and react differently to the same things.

**In Your Mind Replace the Word Calorie with Energy**
Everything we eat contains energy; it is fuel for our body that needs to be used up. Think of food in terms of energy not calories.

**Food Is Hard Work**
Why do you want to carry so much more than you can take? Do you like to pile up tons and tons of work on your

desk, so you have to stay up all night working or on your weekend? Your body is just like you, and it cannot escape from the workload you are giving it, just like you cannot escape from your work or your boss's demands.

## Love Food in a Healthy Way
If you love something or someone too much, in an abnormal way, it is unhealthy. We all love food, but surely we should not go out of our center for it. Remain in control.

## Constructive Complaining
If you complain about a meal you have just started eating because you noticed that it has no salt, too little salt, or for any other reason, the moment you do that, you will not enjoy your meal at all, and the person who made it will feel bad. Let your complaint be used to learn and do better the next time, and be thankful in your mind and think, *I will eat the meal and enjoy it just the way it is*, and you will.

## Enjoy Food for What It Is
Food is a high. Each and everything we eat has an effect on the body and brain. Orange juice gives you vitamin C and boosts your immune system. Apples are excellent detoxifiers, and apple juice can destroy viruses in the body. Bananas and tomatoes contain serotonin, a chemical you already have in your brain that makes you feel happy and relaxed. Beans are high in protein, are beneficial to those with diabetes, and help lower cholesterol. When you eat a meal of beans, your energy level after a few hours is doubled.

*Tip: Add a little cumin powder to dishes containing beans; it prevents post-meal gas.*

So learn to benefit from foods and use them depending on your mood and your schedule. When you eat white sugar in sweets or cakes, you also get a temporary boost of energy; however, if you overeat any of the above, you will not feel this boost, as it will have a reverse effect on you, and keep in mind that brown or raw sugar are better than white. Sometimes when your body has burned a lot in the previous few days, your mind will trigger a desire for an oily or fatty meal such as pizza, and you will enjoy every slice of it without the guilt. But I am sure that logically, your healthy body will never ask you for pizza on a daily basis.

Naturally, people get bored of things; use that as a positive trait and stay balanced instead of only eating healthy or only eating unhealthy.

**The First and Last Cucumber Story**
My mother once told us this story relating to food.

In her youth, her father would buy food in large quantities to feed his huge family of 13 children, and her favorite treat was cucumbers, so when the truck would deliver the groceries, she would take the entire bag of cucumbers and start eating them one after the other until they were finished. She said that after doing this a few times, she realized that the tastiest cucumbers were always the first one, and the last one, and all the cucumbers in between had barely any taste, so what was the point of eating so many in between?

I found this to be true, and noticed that it could apply to anything tasty.

**Hitting the Spot**
While eating a meal, you are looking for that feeling that will make you think to yourself, *Okay, I have had enough, I feel full, I can get up now.* Sometimes, this feeling of "hitting the spot" does not come even though your stomach is fully loaded with food.

I believe that food must be cooked with enough spices, herbs, or other things that make it taste good, and that is not necessarily butter or oil. Sometimes, a meal could be missing just a squeeze of lemon to cause you to feel that the taste *hits the spot*, or perhaps a tiny pinch of salt or chilly could transform the taste, so start learning how to make your food taste better without adding too much of the heavy things.

## It Is Okay to Eat from Several Dishes

Though we have been told in the past not to eat different dishes together because it is fattening, I have discovered that we get the feeling of *fullness* more from *tasting* food than from *quantity*. So for example, if you eat two meals with the same quantity and same amount of calories, on two separate occasions, where one meal has more variety and the other was just one course, you will feel more full and satisfied from the meal that had a variety of tastes. It may take longer to digest, but you will be okay since you have decided to eat your next meal when hungry. Of course, you will not have this luxury at every meal, but it is nice to do that whenever you have the chance.

Have you ever wondered why when you eat with other people, food tastes better? In the presence of other people, you tend to eat more slowly because you feel shy about stuffing your face too fast. When you gulp food, you do not taste it properly, and that is why you keep gulping more, thinking that the quantity will make you full.

Do you ever eat so fast and so much that the mouthfuls do not taste like anything anymore? If you have stopped tasting your food, have a sip of water and then switch to eating something else, like salad; then you can come back to the main course you were having. Make the bites you take into your mouth smaller; that way, eating dinner or lunch will take more time for a smaller quantity. Appreciate the creativity there is in food and the many options man has created along the way.

## "A Big Meal Is Like a Thick Log of Wood"

My husband once said there are meals and drinks you consume that keep you energized for many hours, and some that do not. For example, a sugary snack or fizzy drink will give you a quick boost of energy, but it will not last for many hours, as opposed to a protein and starch meal, such as chicken with pasta and tomato sauce, which will keep you energized for many hours. He compared it with wood for a fire: kindling wood is used to start a fire, and thick pieces of log are required to keep the fire burning for long hours. Think of your energy as the fire and food as the wood.

Obviously, if you place a massive piece of wood on the flame, you will put the fire out completely.

## "Eat to Live; Do Not Live to Eat"

We all love food, but we should not obsess over it and base our entire day around what to eat, and eat at any occasion, even during the times when we ought to be in *burning* mode. There are so many more important and enjoyable things to do.

I am not saying that you should not plan your meals; just do not make your entire schedule about food. Look at the big picture; food is just for your survival, hence the saying "Eat to live."

Revolve your energy around your life's purpose. If you do not have a purpose in life, create one. For inspiration read a book called *What Can You Do To Help Our World?* by Barbara Wolf, Founder of *Global Meditations Network,* and Margaret Anderson. It shows numerous humanitarian organizations around the world that were created by people who like to help others.

\* \* \*

# 2

# PRINCIPLES

Learn The Principles of A Great Body to Keep the Weight Off

Just like the principles of baking are important to the success of baking a cake, the principles of a great body are important to the success of creating and keeping a great body.

If you have never baked a cake, ask someone who has and they will tell you that you cannot succeed in baking a cake, without following the baking principles such as: put a pinch of salt or vanilla in the cake batter in order to avoid rancidity, rub butter on the pan and add flour before adding the cake batter so that the cake does not stick to the pan, do not open the oven while the cake is baking so that it keeps rising, and so on.

The following principles help you to stay within the formula so memorize them and stick to them. If you break them occasionally, do not feel bad; keep yourself in good spirits; that is the point of having a great mind and body.

# Principles of Eating

- ### *No to Deep-Fried*
  The problem with deep-fried food is that the nutrients and vitamins disappear from whatever you fry, and the fat level rises, so you do not get much energy in return. There are far better ways of cooking that will make the food taste really good and will give your body plenty of nutrients and vitamins, including stir-frying, grilling, steaming, and sautéing.

  Once you start your workouts, you will automatically not want to have deep-fried because your mind knows how much effort it requires to burn off, and subconsciously, you will begin avoiding those foods.

  If you really feel like having them occasionally or end up at a friend's dinner and fried food is served, you can eat, as long as it is not more than once or twice a month, and as long as they are placed on a kitchen towel to drain the oil. The best thing is to inform your friend a day before his/her dinner that you do not eat deep fried food.

- ### *Tasty Sauces*
  Sauces are important; they complement the boring taste of certain vegetables or fruits and transform them into something ravishing. The easiest way to make a sauce tasty is to add butter to it; however, that is not the best way. Get into spices and herbs; they give a more unique flavor than butter. Be creative and add honey, maple syrup or jam as a twist. If you require a delicious sauce as a condition to eating vegetables, I say go ahead.

- ### *No to Burnt Barbecue*
  Start grilling over a fire after the flame has diminished and the pieces of charcoal have turned from black to

red-hot, and do not burn the food. (If you have a gas grill this does not apply).

- **Cook with Little Oil, Shortening, or Butter**
  There are many new pans you can buy that do not require a lot of grease to cook food. Train yourself to use the least amount possible of oil, shortening, or butter. What makes something taste good is not fat; it is spices, sauces, herbs, lemons, vinegar, and much more.

  *Hint: Look at your dish, if the oil forms a circle around your meal, this means that you are putting too much oil in your cooking, so reduce the amount next time.*

- **Do Not Overheat Grease**
  When starting to cook make sure you heat the oil for a short time, especially olive oil and butter. Heat the pan a lot, and then add the grease. Wait two seconds, and add in the food immediately after that.

  *Tip: If you cook over high fire because you are in a rush, the meal will not taste as good as one that was cooked over a lower fire.*

- **Less Dry Foods**
  Do not eat too much dry or salty food consecutively in a day, such as pizza, followed by a French bread sandwich, followed by French fries, because it dehydrates you and blocks your digestive system; instead, have fruits, vegetables or soups and water in between those meals, to balance. (Check *Chapter 3*).

- **No to Fake Sugar**
  Avoid drinks and sweets with fake sugar. It is a chemical that your body does not recognize. It is better to have the energy from real sugar to burn other things than to

have something unfamiliar to the body that does not give you energy.

The other reason is because artificial sweeteners raise your sweetness level so your desire for that sugary taste will remain high, and that defeats your aim of trying to bring down the level of sugar you eat.

- ***Replace Cans with Glass/Plastic Containers or Use Frozen or Fresh Food***
  The best option is fresh organic vegetables, but if you have no choice, then it is better to go with frozen over canned vegetables and fruits to avoid metal corrosion, build up of bacteria, and the large amount of preservatives added to the food in cans.

- ***Hours between Meals: Five to Eight***
  Count the hours between meals instead of following the common lunch or dinner hours. For instance, many people eat lunch because it is *lunchtime* even if they do not feel hungry. Waiting five hours between meals is ideal, and you can go up to eight hours; it really depends on what you ate during your last meal.

- ***Eat When Hungry***
  Eating three medium-sized meals a day is best, but if you do not stay on this track then use your hunger as a guide. Do not eat if you are not feeling hungry, even if you have to skip a meal. It is not about what time it is or where you are. Besides, you will enjoy the taste of food more when you are hungry.

- ***Absolutely No Binging***
  This is the biggest principle. You can eat a few chips and a bit of chocolate, but do not go to extremes. Besides, since you are allowed to have whatever you feel like, you will not want to attack food and binge. If you have

this problem now, think to yourself, *This is something I do not ever want to see myself doing.* With time, the habit will go away. Be patient.

- **Do Not Eat Sweets after Each and Every Meal**
  Sweets are a treat; if you have them after each meal they will not feel special anymore and will become a routine that is forced. Have sweets when you are really craving them, therefore, have them randomly and not regularly, and do not have them when you are super full from a meal because you will not enjoy them as much. Learn to wait for things.

- **Eat Before Shopping at the Supermarket**
  If you shop for food on a full stomach, you are more likely going to choose the healthy ingredients you have written on your shopping list instead of buying junk food.

- **Avoid the Supermarket Aisles that Display Chips, Chocolates, and Junk Food**
  At the supermarket, the perimeter is where all the fresh food and produce is displayed, stick to those lanes and avoid the inner aisles stacked with chips, chocolates, and cookies. That way you will not even be tempted at all, believe me, it works.

- **Bites Should Be about a Tablespoon in Size**
  While eating, do not fill your entire mouth and the pockets of your cheeks with food because you will swallow half of it without proper chewing. Fill up your mouth with just *one* tablespoon *at a time* and chew your food thoroughly to help get it digested faster and, in turn, out of your body faster. Also, with smaller bites, you will enjoy the taste of the food more, leaving you feeling content from the meal.

My maternal grandfather who was a doctor, may his soul rest in peace, used to take his time at the dinner table, sometimes chewing a bite of meat up to 50 times before swallowing it.

## Principles of Drinking

- ### *Keep "Drinking" Water around You Always*
  Keep a bottle of water at your desk, next to your bed, next to the TV, and in your car (only in winter time so avoid drinking from a plastic bottle that has been in the sun in your car). If the bottle is not around, you will not drink. It is rare that you will go fetch one; instead, you will let your body get dehydrated.

  After any experience such as shopping, exercising, or a drinking night, you need to replenish your body with water. This is to avoid dehydration and blockages in your digestive system.

  I noticed that some people avoid drinking water when in public areas, as they fear having the urge to go to the toilet when there are none around. So make sure you know where the toilets are.

- ### *Avoid Drinks during Meals*
  Combining beer or water with a plate of food will stretch your stomach. Continued stretching of your stomach will cause it to expand, meaning you will need to eat more and more to fill it up, in turn, giving you a bigger belly. Beer is best on its own or with some nuts and carrots before you eat the meal or at least an hour after you finish eating.

- ### *Avoid Drinks Directly after Food*
  In general, after a meal, and especially if you are super full, avoid drinks, because they will increase the volume

of the food you ate and expand your stomach—and this is something we agreed to avoid.

You can have water, tea, or coffee 45 minutes after food. If you really feel like something right away, have a shot of espresso, tea or white coffee; they help with digestion and are served in a small quantity. To make white coffee, add a drop of orange blossom liquid to hot water without sugar.

- *If You Feel Like Eating Sweets, Drink Water First*
Often times, when you crave sweets, it is in the afternoon or a few hours after your main meals. Instead of rushing to get sweets, drink water first as a test; if water is was what your body needed, then you will not want to eat sweets anymore. If after drinking water, you still feel the craving for sweets, then go for it, or have a light healthy snack such as a handful of dried almonds, fruits or chamomile tea.

- *Avoid Caffeine Products after 5 P.M.*
Some people are lucky that the caffeine found in most chocolates, fizzy drinks, coffees, and teas does not affect their sleep. However, many cannot sleep easily and tend to wake up in the night, especially after eating a large piece of chocolate cake before bed.

# Principles of Your Body

- *Pull Your Belly Muscles 50 Percent Inward*
Keep your belly muscles pulled 50 percent inward as often as possible to prevent them from bulging out, especially while walking and exercising. Having a good posture makes this easier.

- ***Pull Your Buttocks Muscles 50 Percent Upward***
  The buttocks muscles are powerful muscles in your body. They pick you up off the couch when you want to get up; they help you while running or lovemaking. You need to keep them stimulated. Pull them upward 50 percent and if they do not feel strong, then start focusing on them during your workouts and find exercises to train them. Your inner thigh muscles and inner knees support your buttocks muscles, so those need to be activated and tight as well. (You can do buttocks flexes while in waiting areas, driving or on your break from work).

- ***Burn More than You Eat***
  This is the most important formula in this book and must be followed consistently. To sum it up, in order to burn, you must be active, skip meals wisely, and burn before you eat.

- ***Never Let Yourself Starve***
  Do not starve yourself, because your energy level will drop. Being hungry for a maximum of two hours is fine.

- ***Digestion Works Best While You Are Awake***
  Avoid sleep right after meals because the food you ate gets stored as fat, and you wake up hungry thinking that you can eat again. If you happen to fall asleep, wake up and have water because that is what you really need. You can also have a piece of fruit or a sweet.

    The reason some people choose to sleep after lunch is for the escape. They want to wake up and find that the problem disappeared and they are not full anymore.

    If you are sleepy after lunch, engage in an activity, avoid sitting on a couch where you might dose off.

    Avoid having a giant dinner right before bedtime, and if it happens, then stay up another two hours at least. For this reason, it is important to eat dinner by 7 p.m., though this may not be possible with some work schedules. Sleeping on a full stomach causes you to:

1.  Wake up hungry in the morning because you stretched your stomach out. As a result, you eat a lot at breakfast and that keeps your stomach large, making you want more large meals, and this cycle continues.

2.  Toss and turn all night to digest and wake up tired. You deserve beautiful, relaxed, and peaceful sleep every night. You need to rest so you will be full of energy to face another working day.

3.  Store food as fat because it is not burned.

4.  Have nightmares.

5.  You may risk getting heartburn especially while pregnant.

You should not go to bed hungry either. It is hard to sleep while hungry, so always make sure you eat something three hours before bedtime, and if you did not have time for that, a banana right before sleep would be good enough to ground you. If you had to skip dinner because you had a heavy lunch, then surely you will not be hungry at bedtime unless you stay up too late. In this case, have a banana and/or yogurt with bread.

- ***Urinate as Soon as You Feel the Need***
  Do not hold your urine in or delay it; that is unhealthy and can cause infections, plus it can slow down the cycle of digestion. The moment you feel it, go to the toilet if possible.

\* \* \*

# 3

# TEXTURE

<u>Understand the Concept Behind Food Texture to Avoid a Dry System</u>

The concept behind food texture is a crucial guideline for having a great body. You want to make sure your divine system is always working perfectly, pumping liquids and solids in and out, and does not get interrupted or blocked by a combination of the wrong meals.

The foods containing more water have the right texture and keep your system running like a clock; all it takes is making sure you have those meals when required.

## Facts and Information

### Fruits and Vegetables Contain Water[3]
Besides being a good source of vitamins, minerals, and fiber, fruits and vegetables contain lots of water. For

---

3 Cooperative Extension Service – UK College of Agriculture, University of Kentucky, KY

example, oranges are 87 percent water, watermelon is 92 percent water, and cucumbers are 95 percent water. Milk, juice, and other beverages also have large amounts of water. Conversely, dried fruits, nuts, grain products, and baked goods generally contain little water.

On the days when you are dehydrated, for example, after a day at the beach, a drinking night, or a long hard day at work, drinking water alone is not enough; you need to eat water-rich foods, such as watermelon, cucumbers, plums, lettuce, and tomatoes. They can help you stay hydrated and keep you feeling full. Natural foods that contain water help your skin stay moist and less wrinkled and will take care of any type of dehydration.

**Vegetables Are Important**
You may not like vegetables. Perhaps your mother or your supervisor in boarding school made you eat them by force, and that is why you have a memory of not liking them. The truth is they can be quite tasteless if not cooked in an appetizing way. Try to rebuild your relationship with vegetables by making them taste really good. Frying them or boiling them is not advised since they will lose most of their vitamins, nutrients, and energy. You can steam, oven-bake, stir-fry, or add them to a salad. Do not overcook vegetables. Once they are ready, add nice sauces such as teriyaki or balsamic vinegar, to make them really enjoyable. Check the recipes in *Appendix 1* for some other ideas.

My parents taught me how to cook vegetables in a delicious way, so I would always prefer to eat them instead of any fast-food meal.

*Note: Vegetarians who eat healthy rarely get sick with colds and flu.*

## On Beach Days, Replenish with Vegetables and Fruits

If you have planned a day at the beach, in the desert, or in any sunny and hot place, do not eat a big meal or something dry before going and especially once you are there.

In the sun, your body expands because of the heat, and you will seem to have a bulgy stomach. On beach days, have a big breakfast and then eat plenty of fruits and vegetables, or take them with you.

The weird thing is that in the sun, your appetite shrinks; it is only at the end of the day that you feel hunger.

It is best to avoid alcohol in the sun because it dehydrates you faster than usual.

Drink plenty of liquids and eat a healthy meal at sunset to reduce the dehydration caused by the sunshine and heat.

## Stop Having Meat, Poultry, or Fish with Each Meal

We have been accustomed to eating meat at every meal, so without it, we feel like we have not eaten anything. Bu if you get your body used to less meat, it will be healthier. Think of yourself as a graceful human being who does not have to kill a living being at each meal to have a full stomach.

The problem with meat and fish is that they are so salty that they cause your body to store water and in turn cause dehydration. Also, a steak can take up to six hours to digest, so it blocks your system. If you do feel like eating steak, make sure you have a salad and vegetables with it to ease digestion. Then, drink lots of water two hours after you eat, and wait at least six hours until your next meal; that way, your system will always flow like an unclogged sink.

If you eat meat dishes twice a day, cut that to once a day. Do not deny yourself completely; sometimes your body craves chicken, fish, or red meat when you are going through a hectic time at work, or when preparing for an event, and requires energy from proteins.

In my home country, Lebanon, we have 25 different types of healthy appetizers as part of our cuisine, and when we eat at a restaurant, by the time the meat and chicken main course arrives, we are often already full from the appetizers.

**Meals That Block Your System Can Be Used Positively**
Your body takes longer to digest and dispose of certain meals, and this can be used positively because you can skip the next meal without feeling hungry, so suppose you ate such a meal at 11 a.m., skip lunch that day. If you have a long drive ahead, you can avoid stopping for food on the way and save time.

Examples:
- Manakeesh (Middle Eastern breakfast pizza filled with cheese, meat, or thyme)
- Kanafeh (sweet cheese sandwich with sugar sauce)
- Hotel buffet or English breakfast (sausage, eggs, croissant, bread, beans, butter, sour cream, etc.)
- Buffet meals
- Large size burgers
- Steaks
- Or any meal that makes you feel full for the next seven or eight hours.

If you had any of these meals at breakfast, skip lunch; if it was lunch, skip dinner; and if it was dinner, skip breakfast the following day or have a light one.

## Think of Food in Opposites

*Think of Food in Opposites so You Can Balance Meals*

| Heavy<br>Burger, Sausage<br>Buffet | Light<br>Salad<br>Sushi |
|---|---|
| **Dry**<br>Croissant, French Bread<br>Pizza | **Mushy**<br>Vegetable Dish<br>Fruit, Soup |
| **Oily**<br>Fries<br>Deep Fried Food | **Watery**<br>Watermelon, Orange<br>Soup |
| **Sweet**<br>Soft Drink<br>Cake | **Salty**<br>Fish<br>Cheese |
| **Contains Little Energy**<br>Pancake<br>Fast Food Meal | **Gives Energy**<br>Oatmeal, Peanut Butter<br>Beans Dish, Leafy Greens Dish |

When you eat from the things listed in the left column, balance it by having something listed in the right column. That is what I mean by eating according to texture. Suppose you ate something heavy; have something light next. If you had something dry, have something moist next to balance your system. Sometimes you can have a dry dish and a mushy one in the same meal.

Lunch, in general, is better when it is medium to light and not heavy; otherwise, you will want to take a nap, and that is not possible during working hours.

Choose the right foods to eat 75 percent of the time (right column), and overall, make sure your entire diet comprises 70 percent healthy and 30 percent indulgences.

When it comes to sweet and salty, sometimes your body needs one or the other to balance itself. For example, you can tell from your craving for sweets that you have had too many salty things lately. Soft drinks should be consumed rarely, never have them daily or at each meal.

Be conscious of what you eat or make, for example crepes are better than pancakes because they have more water and milk making them less dry on your system. Plus you can add cheese, turkey and vegetables as toppings as opposed to just maple syrup.

## How to Handle a Dry or Oily Meal
If you wake up and find that breakfast is going to be dry, oily, or heavy, such as a croissant, a French bread sandwich, toast, home fries, or fried *Paratha* (a type of Indian pita bread), take precautions by drinking water before the meal, and accompany it with tomatoes, cucumbers, a salad, or fruits. Drink lots of water one hour after you finish eating to flush the meal out of your system. Drink water every 40 minutes until you feel good and do not require any more liquids. Water dissolves foods and fats and keeps your salt and sugar levels low.

You can also have fresh pineapple, or chamomile/jasmine/mint/green/iced tea to replenish your system. Tea, coffee, alcohol, and manufactured beverages are not desirable substitutes for the purely natural water needs of the body. These beverages contain dehydrating agents. They get rid of the water they are dissolved in plus more from the body's reserves.

## Invest in a Juice Maker
There are juice makers for carrots, apples, pineapples, vegetables and more. Invest in one, and make your own

fresh juices because they contain natural sugar, whereas juices purchased from the market have lots of processed sugar in them. You and your health are worth the money spent, and you are fortunate if you can afford to treat yourself this good.

Once in a while you can buy a fresh cocktail juice or a smoothie from a juice bar; they replenish your vitamins naturally.

* * *

# 4

# WATER[4]

Learn When and How Much to Drink to Replenish Your System

*Thirst and hunger give the same rumbling feeling in the stomach; the only way to tell them apart is by drinking water first. If the rumbling feeling is gone, it means you were thirsty; if you remain hungry, it means you must eat.*

—Advice from a survey respondent

4 Some of the information in this chapter was derived from the following sources:
www.shapefit.com/water-benefits.html
www.mayoclinic.com/health/water/NU00283
http://natureheals.hubpages.com/hub/water-cure
http://www-cgi.cnn.com/HEALTH/library/NU/00283.html
http://www.musclemagfitness.com/health-and-medicine/hot-topics/
This One Nutrient Can Improve Athletic Performance, Help You Lose Weight, Look Younger, Written by Jeff Behar, MS, MBA

Water is vital for the body. It makes up 70 percent of the brain, 90 percent of the lungs, and about 83 percent of the blood. Water makes up, on average, 60 percent of the body's weight. The health of every cell in the body depends on water, as does that of every system in the body.

**Water Benefits**
Water is crucial to your health; observe the numerous health benefits:
- Keeps the heart healthy
- Helps digest food
- Transports waste out of the body
- Keeps your large and small intestines lubricated
- Controls body temperature
- Prevents saggy skin
- Assists the body in releasing fat and helps in weight loss
- Helps to dilute potentially harmful substances and chemicals that bombard us daily in the atmosphere so they are not as concentrated in our bodies and flushes them out of our system
- Releases toxic substances from the body, like uric acid and urea, as well as excess sodium
- Flushes toxins out of vital organs
- Prevents diseases
- Reduces the chances of kidney and urinary tract stones
- Keeps joints lubricated
- Prevents and reduces the severity of colds and flu
- Helps to prevent constipation
- Helps to reduce cholesterol
- Helps people with some types of kidney, liver, adrenal, and thyroid diseases
- Provides a moist environment for ear, nose, and throat tissues
- Carries nutrients to your cells
- Is crucial in breastfeeding and pregnancy

- Metabolizes and transports the carbohydrates and proteins that our bodies use as food in the bloodstream
- Helps to promote mind-body fitness

Without the proper flow of water internally, the body will not be able to carry out its functions normally. It becomes drained and tired easily. Just imagine if you do not take a bath every day; dirt accumulates on your skin and makes it look dull, dark, and unhealthy. Your skin becomes itchy, and you develop rashes or, worse, skin lesions. This is also true of the inner organs. When the body is deprived of water, it eventually develops diseases that may become life threatening if left untreated.

The cells in our bodies are full of water. The excellent ability of water to dissolve so many substances allows our cells to use valuable nutrients, minerals, and chemicals in biological processes. Brain function takes priority over all other water dependent systems. The brain is one-fiftieth of the total body weight but receives 18 to 20 percent of blood circulation.

*Tip: Add two teaspoons of freshly squeezed lemon or limejuice to your water. It will help your digestion. The juice will help alkalize your body and neutralize acids created from digesting certain foods or normal cellular metabolism.*

**Water Intake**
Drink as much as you need depending on how active you are, the climate, your health status, and whether you are pregnant or breast-feeding.

Exercise and some illnesses such as fever, vomiting, and diarrhea, cause your body to lose fluids. To replace those fluids drink more water or oral rehydration solutions such as Gatorade, Pocarisweat, or Powerade, these contain electrolytes that can help replenish the nutrients your body needs.

Every day, you lose water through sweating—noticeable and unnoticeable—exhaling, urinating, and bowel movements. Your lungs expel between two and four cups of water each day through normal breathing and even more on a cold day. If your feet sweat, there goes another cup of water. If you make half a dozen trips to the bathroom during the day, there go six cups of water. If you perspire, you expel about two cups of water—and that does not include exercise-induced perspiration.

For your body to function properly, you need to replace this water daily by consuming beverages and food that contain water.

*Women* need roughly 2.2 liters per day (about 9 cups).
*Men* need roughly 3.0 liters per day (about 13 cups).

Do not choose the nighttime to drink all your required liters, because you will not be able to finish them all in one sitting, and you will disturb your sleep by having to wake up during the night to use the toilet, so it is better to drink them throughout the day.

*Research results about Water Consumption:*
- 42 percent drink during a meal and that is not encouraged.
- 60 percent drink after a meal and it is best to drink one hour after the meal.
- 70 percent drink when they wake up on an empty stomach and that is good.
- 34 percent drink before a meal and that is highly recommended though it does not seem to be very popular among people.

## On Dehydration

A person would have to lose 10 percent of his/her body weight in fluids to be considered dehydrated, but as little as 2 percent can affect athletic performance, cause tiredness, and dull critical-thinking abilities. When dehydration occurs, it means that you do not have enough water in your body to carry out normal functions. Even mild dehydration can sap your energy.

Water is the primary substance and the leading agent in the functions that take place in the human body. The lack of water in physiological situations has been associated with disease conditions like asthma, hypertension, ulcers, allergies, and arthritis.

Dehydration poses a particular health risk for the very young and the very old. Signs and symptoms of dehydration include:

- Excessive thirst
- Fatigue
- Headache
- Dry mouth
- Little or no urination
- Muscle weakness
- Dizziness
- Constipation
- Light-headedness

## Cure Constipation

Water does not solve constipation on its own, even though constipation is sometimes caused by lack of water. It helps a lot though.

When the body gets too little water, it takes what it needs from internal sources, and the result is dehydration. But when a person drinks enough water, normal bowel function usually returns.

Constipation can block your system. It is a sign that you may have been eating dry foods. As a result, new food intake gets piled up and may be stored as fat; it may also lead to a bulgy stomach and leave you feeling uncomfortable and moody. What is worse is that constipation may cause hemorrhoids.

There are many easy remedies to cure constipation and have your system working normally again. For example, start your day with a high-fiber cereal, cucumbers, grapes, or dry fruits on an empty stomach, followed by lots of water for the first few hours of the day. If you have spent days eating sandwiches and pizza, your system can recover with one big chicken and vegetable soup. Sometimes, constipation can happen after you ate a series of small meals; eating a big meal may help your constipation by pushing out the digested food in your system. The main idea is never to get constipated in the first place.

**Thirst Is Not Always a Reliable Sign**
If you are healthy and not in any dehydrating conditions, you can generally use your thirst as an indicator of when to drink water. But thirst is not always an adequate indicator of your body's need for fluid replenishment. The older you are, the less you are able to sense that you are thirsty.

Wherever you go, carry a full water container with a secure lid and continually drink throughout the day to stay hydrated.

**Diabetes—Staying Safely Hydrated**
Make a conscious effort to keep yourself hydrated and make water your beverage of choice. Nearly every diabetic adult should consider doing the following:

Take water breaks instead of coffee or tea breaks.

At social gatherings substitute alcoholic drinks with sparkling water.

## Water Helps to Reduce Fat and Water Retention

Water suppresses the appetite naturally and helps the body to metabolize stored fat. Studies have shown that a decrease in water intake will cause fat deposits to increase, while an increase in water intake can actually reduce them.

The kidneys cannot function properly without enough water. When they do not work to capacity, some of their load is dumped onto the liver. One of the liver's primary functions is to *metabolize stored fat* into usable energy for the body. But if the liver has to do some of the kidneys' work, it cannot operate at full throttle. As a result, it metabolizes less fat so more fat remains stored in the body and weight loss stops. Since we know that water is the key to fat metabolism, it follows that the overweight person needs more water.

Drinking enough water is the best treatment for fluid retention. When the body gets less water, it perceives this as a threat to survival and begins to hold on to every drop. Water is stored in extracellular spaces (outside the cell). This shows up as swollen feet, legs, and hands. The best way to overcome the problem of water retention is to give your body what it needs: plenty of water. Only then will stored water be released.

If you have a constant problem with water retention, excess salt may be to blame. Your body will tolerate sodium only in a certain concentration. The more salt you eat, the more water your system retains to dilute it. But getting rid of unneeded salt is easy; just drink more water. As it is forced through the kidneys, it takes away excess sodium.

Water helps to maintain proper muscle tone by giving muscles their natural ability to contract.

It also helps to prevent the sagging skin that usually follows weight loss; shrinking cells are invigorated by water that plumps the skin and leaves it clear, healthy, and resilient.

*Note: Fresh fruit juices or vegetable juices count as
a glass of water, as do unsweetened herbal teas.*

## Use New Bottles of Water or Wash Your Bottle Frequently

Every time you drink with your mouth against the bottle,
bacteria from your mouth contaminate the water in the
bottle. If you use a bottle repeatedly, make sure that it was
designed for reuse. To keep it clean, wash your container
in hot, soapy water or run it through a dishwasher before
refilling it or replace the bottle often.

## Hot and Humid Weather Causes Water Retention

If you have just moved to a hot and humid climate, you will
find that the first year you may gain weight due to water
retention, from seven to ten kilos (twenty two pounds) to
be precise.

Relax; this is only normal and temporary. Wait until the
first year passes, and with the help of exercise, your body
will revert to its normal weight.

## Sip Water; Do Not Gulp It

If you gulp water from a glass or a bottle, you consume
mostly air and feel bloated from all the air in your stomach.
When you drink through a straw or sip without gulping
bubbles, you consume 95 percent water; you can drink four
times as much before you feel full.

## Warm and Cold Water

Room-temperature water is easier to drink without hurting
the teeth. It just flows right into the body and helps digestion,
so it is best to have it before a meal or a while afterwards.
Cold water prolongs digestion by solidifying fat in the food
you ate so do not drink cold water directly after a meal.

On the other hand, cold water is refreshing, can help perk you up when you feel sleepy, and causes the body to expend extra energy in order to match the normal body temperature. Therefore, it is best to drink soup or room-temperature water around meals and bedtime, and cold water on its own.

*Tip: Ask for room-temperature water at restaurants.*

**Smoking Darkens the Water inside You**
When you smoke, the water in your body is polluted with nicotine and tar and gets dark. Your blood circulation slows down, and this makes you feel colder than non-smokers during the winter, and slows down your digestion.

Smoking is the opposite of living. Living is breathing pure air to live; smoking is inhaling a harmful substance that decreases your oxygen and your days alive.

If you have tried quitting smoking successfully on many occasions but fell back into the habit, what you can do for now, instead of quitting cold turkey, is cut down to five cigarettes per day, and instead of starting early in the morning and having plenty of cigarettes, start in the afternoon or evening because each cigarette you smoke is followed by an urge to smoke 20 minutes later.

# When to Drink Water

**Always Drink before You Eat Anything, Anything at All**
Food absorbs the water in your body from your cells, and this thickens the blood. If you are not a disciplined drinker, your body will experience minor dehydration and you will feel tired. This is the main reason people feel uneasy after a meal and they end up thinking it is from overeating.

Even if you are not thirsty, drink at least one glass of water before any meal, snack, or dessert, especially if you know that it will be heavy or dry. This will prepare your system for smoother and faster digestion without using water from your cells. The meal will dilute easily and run smoothly through your body, and will be flushed out and less likely to block your system. If your system is dry or dehydrated because you did not drink, then food will stick and take a longer time to move about, and you might feel too full to drink after the meal and may risk expanding the size of your stomach.

*Note: Drinking before food is easier than afterwards. The water has more space to flow right in, and every bite gets plenty of water to dilute it, as opposed to water trying to dilute an entire lump of food.*

**Drink during the Night**
Sometimes your system will wake you up in the middle of the night because it requires water. It would be good to have a bottle of water beside your bed to help digestion and transport waste out of the body.

**Drink Two Hours before Sports**
Drink two glasses of water two hours before doing your workout. If you forget, then take small sips during your workout just to eliminate the feeling of thirst in your mouth, but do not drink a lot while exercising.

Before endurance events have a sports drink rather than just water to replenish the sodium lost in sweat.

**Drink after Shopping**
You will find your body loses water during shopping for clothes, furniture, or food because you walk around so

much. The trick is to always have access to water after the spree is over.

## Drink during Travel

You get so thirsty during travel, but you do not realize it. Always keep a small bottle, ideally two, in your bag, because they will only serve you a cup on the flight, and that is not enough. I would suggest buying that water at the duty-free shop of the airport, since security checks nowadays confiscate bottles containing liquids from your hand luggage.

For a three-hour flight, 500 milliliters (17 oz.) is good; for a flight longer than four hours, one liter (34 oz.) is good. Even if it is just a half-hour flight, you need water because you walk distances and carry luggage.

When you are on a trip abroad, you will walk around a lot from place to place for business meetings, while visiting great monuments, shopping, skiing, or going to the beach. This means you will be burning a lot of energy and fat, so carry water with you and drink plenty.

*Note: The only downside is the lack of toilets during travel, especially road trips.*

## Drink Water if You Feel Like Sweets

As mentioned in the *principles*, drink water before going to sweet things.

The urge for sweets usually kicks in during the afternoon, when your blood sugar drops. This is normal because your body has lost most of its water in digestion; plus, it is nearly the end of the day and you are getting tired from work, so your body will ask for a kick of sugar. Since water is what you really need, it is better to go for that in order to avoid the habit of eating sweets daily; after you drink, you might not want sweets anymore, and if you do, have a small amount.

## Drink Healthy Tasty Water

Read the labels on waters and avoid the ones with high sodium content because they cause water retention.

Check for the PH levels of drinking water, anything above a PH of 8 is good for you.

If you do not enjoy the taste of the water you are drinking, then you are less likely to drink the quantities your body needs. If you need to buy bottles of water instead of using the tap water in your area because it is unfit for drinking, then go for that option, you are worth the investment. If your tap water is fit for drinking but does not taste good, then buy a tap water filter.

If you do not like plain water, buy water that is flavored, or make your own by adding a bit of juice to your bottle.

\* \* \*

# 5

# EXERCISE

Prepare Yourself Mentally to Begin Working Out Twice a
Week for Life

*Those who think they have not time for bodily
exercise will sooner or later have to find time for
illness.*

—Edward Stanley, former Prime Minister of the UK

Exercising cannot be missed; there is no excuse for
avoiding this natural medicine. Strength of mind and body
are equally important. Some of you may have big problems
that you are dealing with and may think of not working out,
but that is the only thing that keeps you stronger than what
you have to deal with in your life. Exercise helps you cope
with stress and catch your breath; activity regulates your
breathing.

In this section of the book, I discuss how important
exercise is for you, while introducing a simple and fun
workout. I am referring to the gym here as the main way to

exercise, even though there are many other things you can do outside the gym if you do not have access to one.

## My Athletic Background

Overall, I am an energetic person and enjoy learning new activities. Throughout my life, my participation in organized sports and work with professional trainers gave me a good knowledge base for proper exercise.

At first, I did not know what to do with myself for an entire hour at the gym, but with time, I created an intense workout plan for an hour followed by a 20-minute swim three times a week. My body was so beautiful and strong then, but eventually, work caught up with me, and I could no longer maintain this routine. There was no way that I could find three nights a week to work out, and I liked my morning sleep so those hours were out of the question, so when I stopped, all the progress I had made started to vanish. It was very difficult to go back to the same level I had reached when I was working out intensively, so I gave up.

One of my discoveries in life is a long-term solution to this problem; and the solution is a less intense workout routine that can always be managed. It took me a while to develop a practical exercise plan that does not make me tired throughout the week and that could be maintained for life. The workout is included in this chapter, so read on and I hope that you will find my method suitable for your lifestyle.

## Benefits of Exercise

- Your metabolism will speed up and you burn all the food coming your way faster.
- Your digestive system will run more smoothly and will seldom get blocked.
- Your body will keep bad cholesterol at a minimum and your veins will stay open and seldom accumulate plaque.

- You will have a healthier and stronger body with which to face life and a powerful immune system to help you fight off diseases and sickness.
- Your muscles will get stronger and support your skeleton better while improving your posture.
- Your skin will become softer and will tighten up as the weight is lost.
- Your brain will release serotonin and endorphins, chemicals that give you a feeling of happiness and help you stay out of depression.
- You will release the tension built up from work and the stress your thoughts cause your body daily.
- Your body will cleanse itself by releasing unwanted elements through sweat.
- You will become a fit and energetic person, and that will make you burn more food that goes into your system.
- Whether you are male or female, stretching, exercise, and Kegels improve your flexibility, endurance and self-confidence during lovemaking because all your muscles are connected, coordinated, and engaged in the experience.
- Exercise gives you enough energy to deal with your daily tasks, and confidence to achieve your life goals and dreams.

Check with a doctor before you exercise if you have any health concerns.

## Mental Attitude
In my research, I was pleased to find that 65 percent of the respondents do exercise and only 35 percent do not. The most often excuse used was, "Too busy, no time," followed by, "Too lazy." Some said they did not like sports or they could not see the results from it. Well, you do not need to see results right away; you need to feel them first.

People get discouraged from going to the gym because they expect immediate and unrealistic results. Please do not go to the gym and count the calories on the machines, hoping that you can remove all of what you ate in one of your meals or what you accumulated over the years.

In a workout you lose between 200 and 600 calories, during that hour only, and are way less than what you consume in a day. It is difficult to count how many calories you lose during the time outside the gym, but surely it is more than what you would lose if you did not work out at all. Even if you burn under 100 calories at the gym, the benefits you reap from working out are the main reason you need to exercise, and it is the most helpful tool to keep you within the formula: *burn more than you eat*.

Make the trip to the gym as important as your trip to work is; it is vital for your survival. The work needs to be done with a positive attitude, and only you can do it.

Before going, envision yourself walking out of the gym after you have finished working out; imagine how happy and fresh you feel. This is a way to motivate you to go in the first place. Think of it as a challenge in your mind and believe you will enjoy the experience. This time is for you and only you, and you deserve it. All aspects of your life will reap the benefits of a fitter you.

**Rebuild Muscles Slowly**
When you have decided to rebuild your muscles, do so slowly and over a long period of time so that you will not injure your joints or muscles, and you will not feel sore after each workout. Feeling sore can discourage you from exercise because it is a painful experience. Do not push yourself out of hatred for stopping, but out of love for your body. It takes time to build a dream, any dream in life. When you reach your goal of being fit, you will feel really solid and happy and you will not regain weight fast.

We lose touch with our muscles when we ignore them for long periods of time. To reconnect with your muscles, your brain will send them electro signals and after a few exercise sessions, they will get reactivated, this is called muscle memory. If you have not been working out for a while, you can expect it will take longer, between three to six months. Keep going and you will eventually get there.

It took me two months to reconnect with my muscles after having been away from the gym for two years. Signs of weight loss began to be visible on my body, and six months later, I was able to reshape certain parts that I set my mind to focus on. However, in the case of my buttocks, the part that needed the most work, it took me two years to reactivate the muscles because I had ignored them most of my life. It also turned out that the inner thighs support the glutes, so those needed strengthening as well.

## The Past Is the Past; Let It Go
Once upon a time, when you were younger, you were thin, nimble and flexible, with tight stretch mark-free and cellulite-free skin. You were full of energy and had free time with fewer responsibilities.

Then life happened to you, and you stopped the discipline of physical activity for many years. Today, you decide to work out again, and you may be trying to reach the same level you were at when you were younger. Be realistic and shape your body to the best of its ability right now, while using another type of workout that suits you.

There are a lot of things you need to let go of on your journey, and learning to detach is a big part of life and growing up. Embracing what comes your way, even if it is gray or no hair is the best way to live.

Some of you swim against the river, as if trying to fight the cycle of life. Going against time and age is literally impossible. Forget before; it is now and tomorrow that counts.

## Decide on a Long-term Goal
You will need to create a goal based on your individual history with exercise and your current fitness level because

we are all different. Assuming that you are starting from scratch, the main goal we must all share is:

*I will work out for the rest of my life for a healthy and strong mind and body. I will not make my outer shape the sole concern.*

To make that goal achievable and sustainable, your exercise schedule should be realistic and comfortable—meaning, it should fit into your busy schedule, complement your life, and the results should not be painful or exhausting.

Three years down the line, once you have rebuilt your muscles, are more confident, and feel that your workout schedule is too easy; it means that you now have a solid base. For a fitter look, you can increase the resistance on machines and use heavier weights to push yourself harder.

If a personal trainer is helping you, let him/her know that you are planning to build your muscles slowly and do not want to pressure yourself from the start. The problem is that a personal trainer will try to get you fit in a short period of time and ask you to workout three to four times a week. Also, he/she will send you home with sore muscles due to high intensity, and that becomes painful and draining. On the other hand, if you are trying to look like a heavyweight champion, then by all means get help to achieve that goal.

The best thing about training with a personal trainer, if you can afford it, is that he or she gives you a different set of exercises each time to ensure that you work out your entire set of muscles.

## The Gym Is Your Best Friend
The gym must be like your best friend. Do you see him or her every day? No, you see your best friend when you have the time. With the gym, go when you can. Twice a week is

ideal. So no more feeling guilty! Make sure your workouts last at least one hour. Go to the gym because you have the time and you want to, not because you have to. Go there to enjoy it and to feel great. Twice a week is easy to maintain, and this way, you will go throughout your entire lifetime, not just an intense six months. This brings me to the most important point. The gym is a must, but not a daily one. As you have tried before, you get into a very tough schedule of workouts and you start going either every day or every other day. Your muscles get so tense, as hard as rocks. If you miss one time, you feel terrible, and sometimes when you miss a few days, you decide never to go again. And then you are back to where you started. Getting very hard muscles will not give your body a nice look anyway; you should build long lean and flexible muscles.

With this in mind, build a new relationship with the gym that will last forever.

## The Best Gym Location Is Near Home

Pick a gym next to your home so that you can work out on holidays and weekends.

If you work seven days a week and want to go to the gym during lunch break, then it would be better to have it next to work. Wherever the gym is, make the trip!

## Easy Does It

Once you are at the gym, do not overdo it. Think of yoga, it is a great way to burn fat in the body, yet it need not be exhausting or strenuous. Focus on your deep muscles and be gentle, there is no need for a painful experience. Be present, conscious and in control of yourself. Remain attentive to your body, parts are blocked and some muscles are strained. If you spend three hours at the gym without focus and talking on the phone it is pointless. Focus on your breathing and enjoy a pleasant full body workout.

The following figure shows that over 60 percent of people already know that their workout need not be too intense.

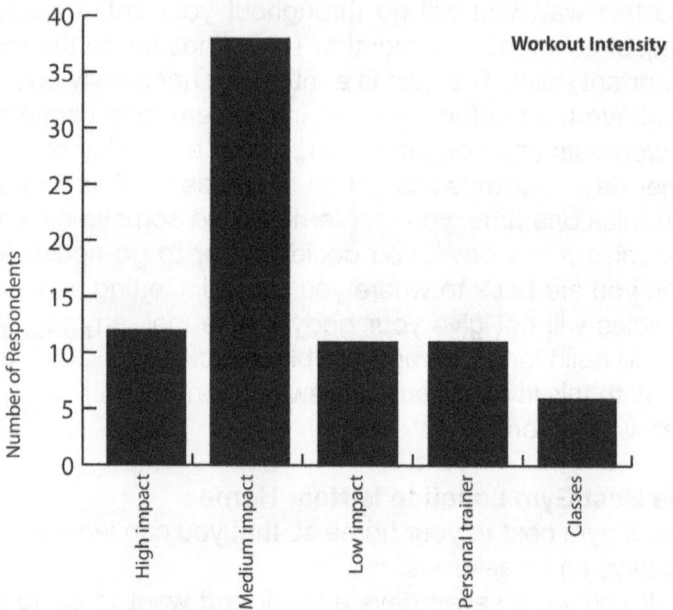

**Brisk Walking instead of Running**
When you restart your workouts, I would suggest brisk walking instead of running during the first two years. Once you get stronger, run for a few minutes during each workout.

While walking, focus on your muscles, think of them, picture them, and connect with them. Let them carry the fat on top of them while heating it to the extent that it melts away like butter.

## Skeletal Muscles[5]

Now, let us talk about the kind of muscle we think of when we say "muscle"—the ones that show how strong you are and let you boot a soccer ball into the goal. These are your skeletal muscles, voluntary muscles that help to make up the musculoskeletal system—the combination of your muscles and your skeleton, or bones.

Together, the skeletal muscles work with your bones to give your body power and strength. In most cases, a skeletal muscle is attached to one end of a bone. It stretches all the way across a joint, the place where two bones meet, and then attaches again to another bone.

Skeletal muscles are held to the bones with the help of tendons. Tendons are cords made of tough tissue, and they work as special connector pieces between bone and muscle. The tendons are attached so well that when you contract one of your muscles, the tendon and bone move along with it.

You have 640 skeletal muscles that come in many different sizes and shapes to allow them to do many types of jobs. Some of your biggest and most powerful muscles are in your back, near your spine. These core muscles help keep you upright and standing tall. They also give your body the power it needs to lift and push things. Muscles in your neck and the top part of your back are not as large, but they are capable of some pretty amazing things. Try rotating your head around, back and forth, and up and down to feel the power of the muscles in your neck. These muscles also hold your head high. Could you imagine your body without your skeletal muscles?

---

5 This information was provided by KidsHealth®, one of the largest resources online for medically reviewed health information written for parents, kids, and teens. For more articles like this one, visit KidsHealth.org or TeensHealth.org. © 1995–2012. The Nemours Foundation/KidsHealth®. All rights reserved.

Relying on only your bones to carry you is not enough. Your muscles carry your bones much better when they are developed; otherwise, you lean on your joints and cartilages, they begin to feel uncomfortable, and wear out as you grow older. Plus, developing your muscles lessens aches in the back, knees, and joints.

Since you now know how your muscles are connected inside, use them.

## Use All Your Muscles, Not Just the Heart

The main reason you need to empower the muscles in your body is to help your heart. Your heart is the most important muscle and you are exhausting it by having it burn all the food you eat daily. To top it off, you have to cope with a heavy workload, a family, or both, so there is so much for your heart to do. Do not expect one muscle on its own to help break down all the stuff you eat during the week, especially with the complexity in food today. Back in the day, food was simpler; now it is mainly processed.

## Stretching Is Vital

Stretching is so important, but cannot work without proper breathing. Stretching after a workout prevents tightness in your muscles, and you become more flexible. You need seven to ten minutes of warm-up before and seven to ten minutes of stretching after skiing, swimming, working out at the gym, or any other activity, and those minutes count as part of the total workout time.

While warming up, stretch the muscles in your neck, arms, waist, hips, legs, back and feet. Do so gently before the workout to avoid tearing your muscles, but at the end of the workout, it is okay to push a little harder because the muscles are more pliable.

## The Reasons You Need to Stretch

- Get into the mood of the workout
- Warm up the muscles
- Avoid exhaustion
- Avoid stiff muscles the day after
- Pump blood in and out of your muscles
- Burn more energy
- Elongate the muscles to create beautiful lean shapes that are not bulky
- Coordinate the whole body
- Tone the body
- Increase flexibility
- Release the energy that was created during the workout, so it can flow to the rest of the body
- Release the carbon dioxide ($CO_2$) that comes from the fat-burning process
- Prepare the muscles for the next workout

The website www.greatbodynodiet.com will have lots of useful information and a section dedicated to stretching.

### Workout Times

The best thing about working out twice a week is that you can always find time for it once on the weekend and once during the week. Make sure there is always a two-day break between your workouts. Anytime during the day is acceptable.

If you work out in the morning before breakfast you will ignite your metabolism, use up stored fat for energy, and feel great the rest of the day. However, if it is one of those lazy days and you woke up hungry and tired, then it would be better to have breakfast to get energized before a workout two hours after breakfast or later during the day.

If you prefer to workout in the afternoon or evening, that is fine too.

*Tip: If you plan to workout after lunch or dinner, wait three hours after eating for best results.*

## Play Chill-Out Music but Not Too Loud

Lounge or chill-out music is preferred throughout your workout or no music. Fast techno beats while you are running. The heart feels the beats and rhythm in a song and then passes them onto other areas.

If you are in a gym and cannot control the music, remember that you are trying to achieve the breath of life and that is a long, deep, and patient breath instead of a short, fast, and shallow one, so do not get carried away by the music or TV screens.

## Substitute the Gym for Other Activities

So you do not like gymnasiums? Fair enough, purchase two DVDs that you can watch at home, one for yoga and one for another activity such as aerobics. Or you can go hiking, running, or swimming outdoors. If the workouts you choose do not have a stretching program, please do an Internet search for some body stretches and follow those.

To avoid getting bored with your two DVDs, include more activities in your life. Gather some friends and play group games like basketball, volleyball, tennis or football. Or you can also learn a new sport, as long as you do something that helps your divine system to function better.

Swimming is good for back pain and posture and helps your body to be more coordinated and burn lots of energy. While swimming, there is no need to go very fast; you are not trying out for the Olympics. Just attempt to reach the other side of the pool however way you can, and do it slowly so that you do not get exhausted from the first two laps. Do not count laps; count the time you spend swimming to know when to stop. Try swimming on your back; it is good for the buttocks and back.

Hiking is great for many things, and mainly for the heart buttocks. When you walk continuously at a reasonable pace, your heart is constantly beating at a higher rate for a long period of time; this is super healthy for your fitness. It is fun to go with friends, your kids, or your partner and connect with nature, let your mind release serotonin and endorphins.

There are trails in most countries around the world. If it is cold outside, dress warm and go hiking. It gives you so much energy; breathing outdoors is good for you.

Surely you have heard of yoga; you might even have tried it. Here are some reminders of its benefits:

- Balances the body
- Aligns the posture
- Decreases stretch marks and cellulite (I was told about this by an Indian yoga instructor, and later on I personally experienced it)
- Increases flexibility
- Improves sexuality
- Reduces fat in the body
- Improves breathing
- Improves concentration
- Relaxes the body and mind
- Strengthens deep inner muscles
- Improves blood circulation
- Releases tension
- Improves metabolism
- Stimulates the organs in the belly area and keeps fresh blood flowing through them

Though yoga is so beneficial, it is not sufficient. I would suggest doing yoga once a week or twice a month, unless you feel you need more of it, along with another workout program once a week.

**Focus to Fix**
Focus on the area that you want to fix in your body, and always be aware of it while you are working out. Do not think of other things or talk to people; just be completely in the moment. For example, you want to fix your back muscles, dedicate lots of exercise to the back area. If you have big hips, do more exercises for that part of the body.

**The Internet Has Every Exercise You Might Need**
Constantly think about the area in your body that you promised to work on, always connect with it, and make sure it is activated the entire time. Go beyond that, and find videos on the Internet that work out that specific area; for example, if you think your inner thighs need work, type "inner thighs exercises videos" in the search box of your browser. You will find lots of links. Add those exercises to your one-hour workout.

> *Try this exercise: while standing up, bend your knees slightly, hold your belly in, put your hands behind your ears, and rotate your upper body from left to right and from right to left, while twisting your waist as if you were squeezing a wet towel. Do it at least 10 times and as often as you can. This helps to melt fat around the waist, giving you a thinner one (see photo 1.0).*

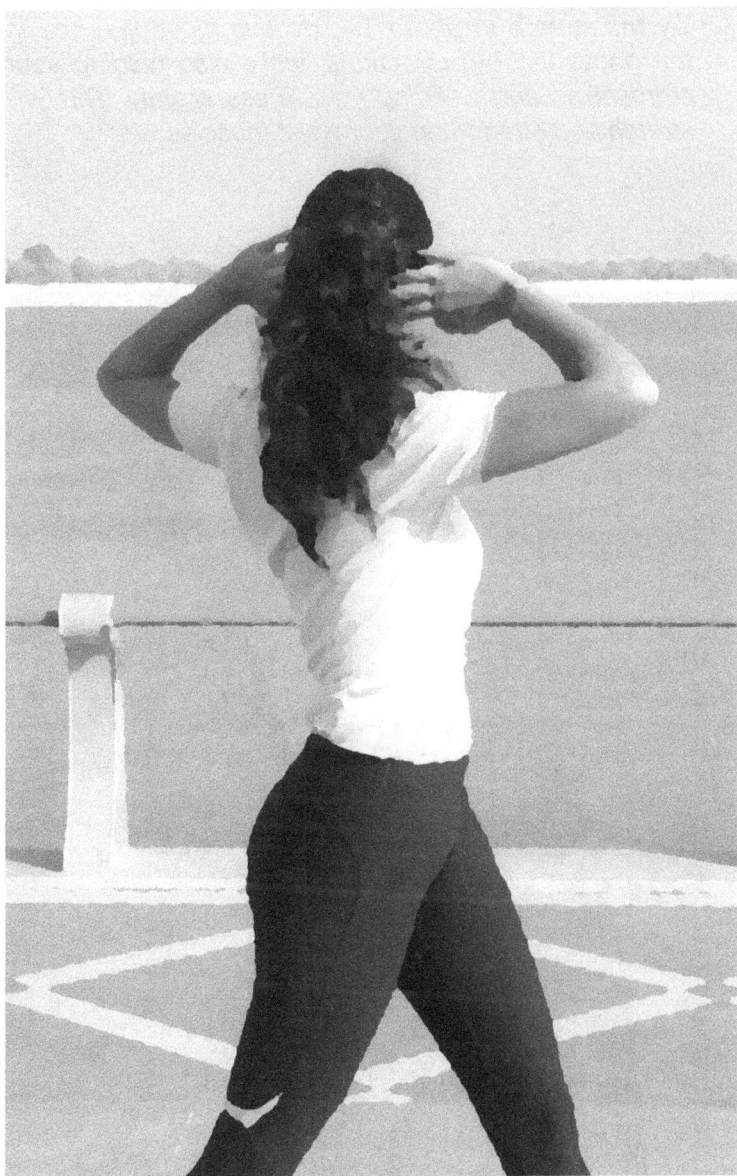

*Photo 1.0, an exercise to shrink your waist size.*

*(Image by Photographer Georges Maroun)*

*Try the stretch in photo 1.1; do this move you see in the photo in both directions, while also holding your stomach in and bending your knees slightly. This will stretch and strengthen your waist muscles.*

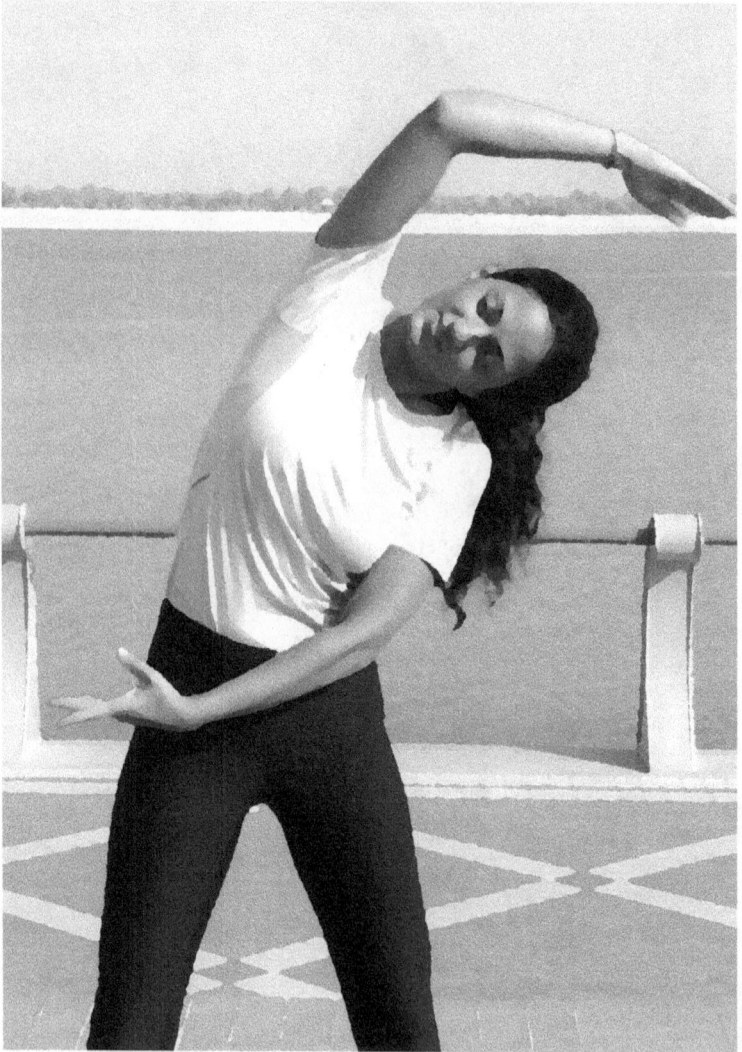

Photo 1.1 (Image by Photographer Georges Maroun)

## During Busy Periods Workout Once for Longer

In general, working out once a week may not be enough to feel fit; however, if you have no other time during the week because of a project, and you only have one day off per week, instead of stopping entirely, use that day to work out at least 90 minutes. The extra 30 minutes can be spent swimming or on machines, with lots of breathing to ease the stress during that busy period of your life. If you do this for one or two months as maintenance for the usual two workouts a week, you will be fine.

If you do not have at least one day off during the week, be careful because you might be overworking yourself, and that can become counterproductive.

## Wait at Least One Hour after Food to Make Love

Making love is a form of exercise (though it is not to be considered as a substitute for exercise), therefore having a full stomach will create discomfort during this pleasurable activity, and so you are better off waiting at least an hour after food.

> *Tip: The Kegel exercise, named after Dr. Arnold Kegel[6], consists of repeatedly contracting and relaxing the muscles that form part of the pelvic floor, now sometimes colloquially referred to as the "Kegel muscles."*
> *These exercises are usually done to reduce urinary incontinence, aid with childbirth in women, and reduce premature ejaculatory occurrences in men.*

## Fresh Air Where You Exercise

If you exercise in a closed room, after 20 minutes the air will become $CO_2$ (carbon dioxide). This stale air will make you

---

6 Wikipedia, s.v. "Kegel exercises."

tired. In order to avoid that, open a window or turn on the A/C on low or on fan mode.

Breathing fresh air is extremely important, as it carries the $CO_2$ out of the body and the $O_2$ (oxygen) into the body to get your blood flowing faster, increase your stamina, and help you digest food faster.

Breathe *slowly, deeply,* and *continuously.*

## Breathe Using Your Full Lung Capacity

We sometimes allow our mood to impact our deep breathing. Learn the following simple way to breathe better using your entire lung capacity.

> *Try it now: slowly exhale to the extreme using your chest muscles and your diaphragm (the muscle in the abdominal area that controls the lungs, also used while singing or performing yoga) until there is not one drop of air left in your lungs and they naturally fill up with air. Repeat the same thing once more by exhaling, and then inhale and continue your regular breathing from there on.*

Most of the time inhale air through your nostrils and exhale from the mouth unless you are doing yoga or cardio where you are better off breathing in and out of your nostrils.

> *Tip: Ladies, do not wear a bra that is too tight and squashes your lungs, because it may impact your breathing.*

## The Medium-Impact Monthly Workout Schedule

The following table is a sample of workouts during the month of February, followed by a table showing two medium-impact workouts, each one is 60 minutes long and can burn around 165 calories. If you manage to do nine workouts per month, every month, for your entire lifetime, it is a lot better than working out four times a week for six months and then quitting entirely. Besides, when you go back to the gym after having stopped for a while and suddenly start going every day, you shock your system and your heart. It needs time to open up the channels again for circulation and the fast pumping of blood. So do it gradually instead and let your body get used to working out again.

## Workout Schedule Excluding Sundays

Skip 2 or 3 Days Between Workouts, You Still Get 9 Workouts in February

| Monday | Tuesday | Wednesday | Thursday | Friday | Saturday |
|---|---|---|---|---|---|
| Feb 1 Workout | | | Feb 4 Workout | | |
| Feb 8 Workout | | | Feb 11 Workout | | |
| Feb 15 Workout | | | Feb 18 Workout | | Feb 20 Workout |
| | Feb 23 Workout | | | Feb 26 Workout | |
| | Mar 2 Workout | | | Mar 5 Workout | |

*Exercise*

# Two Workout Samples One in a Gym and One Outdoor
Each Workout Is Sixty Minutes, and Burns Approximately 165 Calories

| | Gymnasium | | | Outdoor | |
| activity | Minutes | Calories | activity | Minutes | Calories |
| --- | --- | --- | --- | --- | --- |
| Warm-up Stretches | 10 | 5 | Warm-up Stretches | 10 | 5 |
| Bicycle Quickstart | 5 | 30 | Walk or Hike | 15 | 40 or 60 |
| Walk Fast Quickstart | 10 | 30 | Cycle or Swim | 15 | 60 |
| Stepper or Glider | 10 | 30 | Squats, Lunges | 5 | 15 |
| Weights, Sit-ups, Lunges | 15 | 60 | Push-ups, Sit-ups, Back | 5 | 15 |
| Cool-down Stretches | 10 | 10 | Cool-down Stretches | 10 | 10 |

95

- If you can swim for 15 minutes after your workout, that is truly a plus and will use up at least 50 additional calories.

- These workouts are all you need for the first three years of getting back into shape; you will not feel bored or anxious because each goal is five to ten minutes long on one machine, instead of one hour of running on the same machine.

**Facial Muscles[7]**

You may not think of it as a muscular body part, but your face has plenty of muscles. You can check them out next time you look in the mirror. Facial muscles do not all attach directly to bone like they do in the rest of the body. Instead, many of them attach under the skin. This allows you to contract your facial muscles just a tiny bit and make dozens of different kinds of facial gestures. Even the smallest movement can turn a frown into a smile. You can raise your eyebrow to look surprised or wiggle your nose.

Knowing that your muscles are connected to your skin helps you in shaping your face, and yes, doing the right facial exercises can leave you looking young. Look for some facial exercise videos on the Internet. While working out, let your facial muscles work out too; they are what keep your face looking young, not creams (all creams can do is keep your skin moist).

> Try this now: Exaggerate a smile, or say these letters out loud: AAAAA, OOOOOO, UUUUUU, EEEEEEEE. Say them a second time but this time with your head dropped to the back and your chin up.

---

7 Facial Muscles from KidsHealth.org or TeensHealth.org. © 1995–2012. The Nemours Foundation/KidsHealth®. All rights reserved.

*Note: In general, a happy and active person will always look younger than someone who is of the same age but is lazy and unhappy.*

Derived from the survey, the following table shows what type of exercise people usually do.

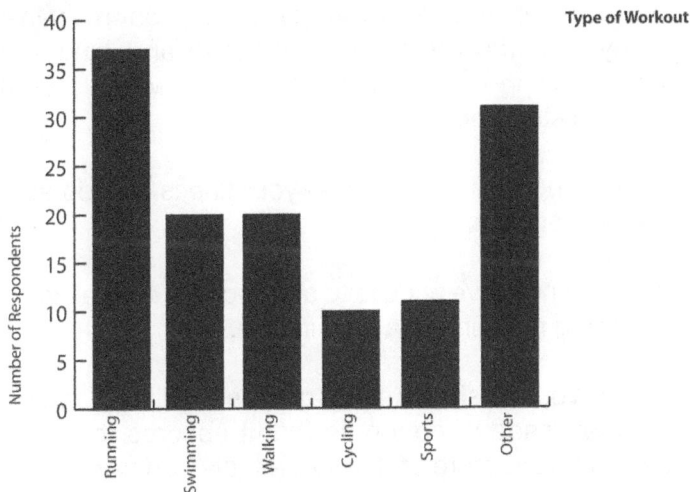

## Useful Tips for Exercise

- Avoid carrying heavy weights in the gym if you have not been working out for a long time. You could injure yourself; take it easy. Besides, carrying light weights and doing slow movements at high repetition is harder to do and is more beneficial in the long term.

- On weight machines, do slow and controlled movements and be sure that during each exercise, you are making a mind-muscle connection.

- If you have not been exercising for a long time, avoid getting into exercise classes that are not beginner level. Check with the instructor on the fitness level of the class before joining it because if it is too difficult, this can directly impact your ability to keep up with the class, and can discourage you from continuing.

- While doing any exercise, especially on machines, always *breathe out* while contracting and *breathe in* while relaxing your muscles. Do this slowly so that the effect is stronger.

- After doing your sit-ups, hug your knees and do some Kegel exercises.

- If you do not have access to a hiking trail, try walking on a running machine at a high incline.

- When you finish working out, immediately wear a sweater made of cotton so that it absorbs the sweat, helps release more of it, and protects you from getting tense muscles or a cold. If you go into the A/C, you will not sweat it out.

- It is best to take a warm shower immediately after you finish working out in order to relax the muscles and continue the fat burning process. Before you take a shower, switch off the A/C or turn on the heat depending on the season.

- Eat protein meals after exercise.

- Avoid eating or drinking anything that contains lactose before a workout.

- Stretch leg or arm muscles a couple of minutes between machines.

- If you do not feel like starting with stretching, do something like cycling or brisk walking for 10 minutes, and then do your warm-up stretches afterwards.

- Buy a yoga mat for floor exercises, like sit-ups, back-ups, and push-ups.

- Take your gym clothes to work; that way, you will feel encouraged to go to the gym afterward.

- Take your gym clothes on business trips; you might find time to work out, and most hotels should have a decent gym with minimal equipment.

- For this lifestyle change to work, you have to understand it, apply it, and believe in it.

- The speed of your breathing must be as fast as your steps, so if you are running, take short, deep, and fast breaths; if you are walking, take long, deep, and slow breaths.

- Remain hydrated at the gym by taking small sips of water when thirsty.

- Do not reach a level where you cannot breathe anymore. It will only make you dizzy. The point is to be moderate, balanced, and conscious of every movement, so that the body and mind are working in coordination.

- If muscles get too hard after a series of tough workouts, it will create a wobble effect because the skin and the muscles will not be acting as one; they will kind of separate. Moderate workouts will create lean muscles and will keep your skin, fat and muscles as one. Later on, when your body is in very good shape and you have lost weight, you can start pushing yourself harder and the wobble effect will not happen.

- Self-discipline is the most important factor, and it is what we work so hard to teach our kids. Remember the discipline your parents and school taught you, and apply it on yourself.

- The chest muscles can be empowered by push-ups, so do 10 during each workout. Once they are stronger, they pull your breasts slightly upwards when contracted.

- Consciously use your buttocks muscles as much as possible while standing up, walking, and going up staircases. Slow, aware movements are always better.

- When you are sick, you are excused from exercise, instead, get plenty of rest.

- My workout was just a suggestion. Build your own program according to what you enjoy doing in the gym.

- People tend to work out the muscles in their bodies that are already dominant and strong. Try to focus on your weak muscles during your workouts; that is the only way you will ever strengthen them.

- Some cultures do not make sports a priority, nor do they give them any importance. Sports should be encouraged in the workplace just as they are in schools; they help create happiness and positive energy, in turn, increasing productivity.

- Do house work. This is the most beautiful way to get cleanliness and tidiness around you, and you get a workout out of it. Every house cleaning activity burns a certain number of calories; you can search for that information on the Internet just to have an estimate.

- Dance! Get warmed up by stretching, play your favorite songs, and spend time just dancing by yourself, in your underwear. Sweat out all that stress, enjoy your body, and be uplifted.

- A useful routine for sit-ups that helps get rid of a belly:

- Do 10 sit-ups, relax, breathe, point your toes, and move your arms up and above your head, in the opposite direction of your pointed toes. Stretch your belly to the max. Let its muscles de-contract while you breathe in slowly and rest. Then do another 10 sit-ups and so on.

- If you ever feel discouraged by your body because it is taking too long to improve, try to see how far you have come, and remember that the surest way to improve is by continuing to work at it; by quitting, you lose everything you have done so far. Keep your focus on the overall lifestyle change, not the pounds and inches. This is about living longer, healthier, fitter, and happier!

- Some people such as the military, athletes, dancers and more, at some point in their life pushed themselves during exercise beyond others and developed their muscles to the maximum. This gives them a strong base long-term and if they were to re-start exercise after having stopped for a long time, they can easily reconnect with their muscles and will do so faster than regular people.

- If you have never developed your muscles to the maximum before, especially while young, it will take you longer to connect with them, but just know that it *is* possible if you stay determined and continue working at it over a long period of time. Before getting fit, everybody starts from scratch. Start moderately, and as you get stronger, increase your resistance. This should feel like an easy climb on a hill, not like a climb on a steep mountain. Good luck!

* * *

# 6

# HABITS

Adopt Easy Habits that Compliment Your Busy Lifestyle

It is not *what* you eat; it is the habit of eating it.

For example, eating sweets after each and every meal is a not a good habit, but eating sweets occasionally is.

Everything you have read so far is about new habits for your lifestyle change; however, there is more for you to learn in this chapter.

Developing these new habits is very easy, because you do not need to make any major changes in your life, just some adjustments here and there. These habits will help you maintain your weight throughout your life, and you will always be in control of it.

## Shopping

### The Food Pie for a Balanced Body
Take a look at the photograph on the cover of the book. Remember this picture when you go for your weekly

shopping at the supermarket, and fill your shopping cart with goods that are 70 percent healthy, and 30 percent other.

The following is the best balance of intake on a monthly basis, whether eating out or at home.

| | |
|---|---|
| Fruits & Vegetables | 30% |
| Proteins & Dairy | 25% |
| Carbohydrates & Fiber | 30% |
| Desserts | 15% |

The meals we cook at home must be mostly either salads or soups, with a main course that contains vegetables and meat.

Fruits are great to have in the morning, two to three hours after a meal, before a meal, or before bedtime.

Cereals, cheeses, croissants, eggs, and bread make a wonderful breakfast, and there is enough time to burn it.

Shopping for fresh food is expensive, but you are worth it. Investing in your health is better than investing in belongings.

Cooking with the best ingredients increases your chances of ending up with a tasty meal.

## Sweets

If you feel like eating a sweet treat, go for it, and sometimes choose fruits over processed sweets and chocolates. The main reason is because our tong gets trained to a certain level of sweetness, do not let that level rise, always bring it back to neutral by having healthy sugars from fruits or nothing at all.

Have you noticed how when you buy a box of sweets and keep it in the cupboard, you only feel like eating it the first day and then the thought of it over the next few days is not as exciting anymore? So do not force yourself to eat it just because it happens to be there. Think: *Waste or waist?*

> *Tip 1: Feel like a heavy sweet, such as a big piece of apple pie with ice cream or cheesecake at dinnertime? Then let that be your dinner.*

> *Tip 2: If you are only two people living together and you bake a big cake, try to send some of it to your neighbor or bake it the night you have friends coming over so that they consume at least half of it, and you and your partner are only left with a few slices instead of an entire cake.*

# Eating

**Moderation Is Balance**

Most things are good in moderation; extreme in anything is not, such as overeating, overdrinking water or alcohol, oversleeping, etc. Better yet, the more you wait for something the more you enjoy it—but do not wait too long because that is extreme.

Finding balance is a tough thing to do. First, you need to know how much of something saturates you; it is different for each person. After you determine this, draw a line before that point. Once you learn where the lines are in every aspect of your life, you will know when to start and when to stop. Envision yourself walking on a rope and trying to achieve balance.

Moderation means not all the time; it means that a habit does not take control of you; it means that you can equally say yes or no to something and have it occasionally, so that you always enjoy the experience and do not get saturated; it means that when you decide to have something, you do not have too much of it.

Moderation is balance because you are not exceeding a certain level; you remain in equilibrium. Moderation keeps you in a zone of wanting something, because you do not constantly have access to it. And if you do not forbid yourself from eating anything, such as sweets, then you will not want those things because you know you have the choice of eating them anytime.

## When You Wake Up, Wait before Eating

When you wake up, do you start your work as soon as you open your eyes? No, you probably need at least 45 minutes before you can begin working with an opened mind.

Your system is the same way; it needs time before beginning to work at digestion. Your stomach is still very tight; so do not expand it with food until you get hungry or until your digestive juices are ready to receive food.

The best way is to get dressed first, drink water, and then eat breakfast; that way, you will have waited at least 45 minutes from the time you woke up. There will be days when you have no time to wait, and you are still not hungry at all. In this case, take the breakfast with you to work and have it when you get hungry, and it will taste so much nicer.

If you wake up late and know that your lunch is in one or two hours, then have lots of water and skip breakfast. As previously mentioned, it is okay to feel hunger sometimes; that is the time when the body is burning the previous meals. Some people eat just because they want to avoid getting hungry later; this should only be done before getting on a plane that does not serve food, or before a long meeting at work, etc.

## When to Stop Eating

If you stop before feeling full, you will not be satisfied; your hunger will linger on, and you will want to eat other things between meals. If you stop when you are too full, you will expand your stomach and feel pain. (Remember the promise you made to treat yourself very well.) It is best to eat your meal slowly and then stop three to five bites *after* the feeling of fullness has occurred.

I once got to a point where my stomach shrank, and I lost so many kilos that I was diagnosed as underweight. People kept telling me that I did not look healthy and that I was too thin. That was not the look I wanted to have. Christmas season came up, and there were lots of dinners and good food, so I started overeating and stretching my shrunken stomach beyond its limit, until I literally felt that something was torn in there and it hurt a lot. After that, every time I ate, that same pain came back, until I realized that the best way to heal this was to stop getting full for a few days. It worked!

If you have been on a spree of overeating for a few days or weeks, do not panic; you can still turn things around. The first step is to cut down on sweets entirely, and lower your intake of food for two to three days. Once you start feeling in control again, you can have normal, balanced meals.

*Tip: Your mind usually calculates the amount your eyes see on the plate before you eat and makes enough space for it before you start; that is why going for seconds is not advisable. Decide on the right amount before beginning the meal.*

*Try this: Open both your hands and put them next to each other, the size of both palms makes a good amount of food on a plate to eat.*

- Ramy G. Ramy

**No Interruptions**
If you put a full load of clothes in the washing machine or all of your dishes in the dishwasher, once you have

pressed the start button, you cannot add anything more to this cycle because it will not get cleansed properly. It is the same with digestion. Once you have filled your stomach with a good meal, wait until you really feel that everything is out of the way. A few hours after you have eaten, your body usually sends a signal when the food has been digested, and it could sometimes be a burp, so follow your instinct on this one and do not kid yourself.

Digestion takes three to seven hours, depending on what you ate. On average, always keep a six-hour gap between meals, and use your logic so as to know when to eat again. Certain fruits and drinks are okay because they will aid in digestion; light snacks as interruptions are also okay sometimes, but do not make it a habit.

> *Tip: Always have your mind made up and your answer ready. For example, you go out with friends for drinks. You have eaten well all day and just had dinner. Your system is digesting, and some alcohol would help to get the blood moving faster and give you a kick to go dancing to burn even more. Your friends decide to order food, and they ask you to eat with them or have a few bites. Politely say, "No, thank you." Your system is already working to digest dinner. Remember, no interruptions.*

### Evade Binging

Feel like taking it out on food? I strongly advise against binging; in fact, this is one of the main *principles*.

If you start binging, catch yourself in *that* moment and remember that it is never too late to stop the spiral simply by deciding to stop. Do not go down that track. Divert your energy to something productive!

**Buffets**

At weddings, corporate events, or any type of event that involves a large, yummy buffet, here is what you can do to make the best of it without expanding your stomach and complaining later. First, drink a glass of room-temperature water and then follow these steps:

1.  Knowing that you are most probably going to eat starters, main courses, and desserts, make your calculations early. Before you get into the queue, have a quick look around at the dishes on display. You might find things you really like, and those are the ones you should select; if you do not look around first, you may stop at each dish and will fill your plate with things you do not like that much, and the space in your stomach will be wasted.

2.  Pour one or two spoonfuls maximum from each starter you like, and once you have sat down, try the different things on your plate. If there is something you did not like because they did not cook it well, then do not eat it. If one of the things you picked was especially yummy, you can go back and take another serving later with your main course. (The main reason you must only take one or two spoonfuls is so you do not throw food away, another reason is so that you can leave enough room for seconds if you discover something yummy.)

3.  While going for main courses, do not take from everything; select only the things you really like and add those in small quantities, because if you overfill your plate, then the dishes mix together and they will all taste the same. At first, take one bite from each type to see which one is the best and focus on that. There is no need to finish your whole plate if you have already reached fullness, because you need to leave the last few bites you are entitled to after fullness for the desserts. Once you are done

with main courses, if there was something you really enjoyed and you still have room for, then perhaps you can go back for another small serving, but if that made you reach your last bite, then you may have to skip dessert.

4. As for desserts, take small pieces of your favorites and have a few bites, but if you really do not have space for them, then skip that part, and next time, manage your first two courses better.

5. A small espresso would be nice to follow, but mainly drink water and chamomile or green tea two hours after this big meal.

After a buffet, do not think of eating anything for at least eight hours, because your body has plenty of work to do. If it was a lunch buffet, then skip dinner that night; if it was a dinner buffet, then forget breakfast the day after.

Occasional buffets are good; because you get all the food types that your body has been missing.

## Eat It until You Cannot Stand the Sight of It

One day, I discovered a new kind of doughnut and fell in love with the taste of it (this rarely happens to me by the way). I kept buying it and eating it every two days until one day, I could not stand to smell it or even see the box. And there, I got rid of the habit of eating it; it was no longer a temptation for me because I felt saturated.

This does not mean that you should eat five boxes at once (remember, no binging). Have it as often as possible in reasonable quantities until you do not want it anymore. The idea is to eat it consecutively, not all at the same time.

I do not encourage this method to be used more than once or twice in your lifetime.

## Eat in the Now

Our senses do not work as well when they are all engaged at the same time.

When you eat, stay in the moment. If you are talking to people around you, working at your desk, talking on the phone, or thinking of something that has upset you, you will not be focusing on eating, and you will not know when to stop or enjoy the experience. Let the food spend time on your tongue and taste it before it goes down to your body.

Chew your food slowly; avoid gulping it down in chunks.

## Eat at a Moderate Pace

The first step in the digestive cycle is chewing. Do not eat too slowly, as your food gets cold and you will not enjoy the rest of it. On the other hand, do not eat too quickly, because it will be more difficult to digest and you will not feel full.

As per the words of a talented American sculptor, Jon Hudson Barlow, "Eating and love-making are two pleasures that must be done slowly to enjoy the experience and make it last."

## If You Are a Parent

If you have children, they will often want to eat sweet or salty things. This is normal; they are discovering new tastes. However, you already know those tastes well, so do not jump in and eat as soon as you see one of your kids eating something, knowing that it is not right for you at this moment or might interrupt your digestion.

For example, you might be on your way to the gym, and your kid opens a box of chocolate wafers in front of you. It is better if you wait until after your workout to have some, if there are any left.

## Subtract Meat

Reduce the amount of meat you intake by occasionally subtracting it from your dishes. For example, if you usually cook okra with meat, subtract the meat and keep the same cooking method and ingredients. There is a saying, "Is the taste in the steak or in the sizzle?" I think that it is in the sizzle. The taste will be just as good without meat, and it is so much lighter on your system.

## Feed Your Friends

While eating with friends, share your meal with them, and you can taste many different dishes, which will ensure that you get full. If some of your friends are not the type to do so because it is not in their book of etiquette, that is okay; save it for those who accept it.

Some restaurants serve big portions, it is an opportunity for two people to share one plate. Share a junk-food meal; you will walk out of the restaurant with a happy smile instead of guilt.

## Eating at a Restaurant

Water must be the first thing you order and preferably at room temperature. You should order healthy meals 70 percent of the time; keep the 30 percent for cravings. Eat according to how full you feel, and if you do not have space, avoid the dessert or share it with someone at the table. Wait at least two hours after dinner before sleeping.

## Practice Self-Restraint

Many religions honor fasting because it is a big sacrifice. It also happens to be a great way to practice self-restraint.

There are different ways of fasting depending on the religion; one is by going without food or drink from sunrise until sunset.

Do not be afraid of fasting a few times in your life, through it you will learn to strengthen your will power in light of almost any temptation that comes your way. Food is the main one—though it really should not be considered a temptation but a blessing.

Your mind orders the yes or no to eating, so if you are strong in the mind, you will be able to resist anything knowing that you are doing the right thing for yourself.

## Fasting Tactics

If you have decided to fast, make sure you drink at least two glasses of room-temperature water while you are having your dates at the time you are breaking the fast. If you do not drink before you eat, you will not have enough space to drink after you eat and will have to wait at least two hours before you can drink properly. You will then feel very thirsty and lethargic the next day while fasting again. Once you finish your meal, wait at least two hours and drink lots of water.

Have a full meal at sunset containing proteins, carbohydrates, and fats such as soup, salad, main courses, and dessert. By 10:00 p.m., you can have a small meal two hours before sleep if you have space in your stomach. If you do not have space, then do not eat anything.

# Self-Talk

## Do Not Hate Yourself If You Overeat

When you overeat—and this should happen rarely—what you can do to jump-start your digestion and deal with the problem instead of blaming yourself is concentrate on your breathing for 10 minutes, breathing deeply and using your full lung capacity.

Or stay seated so that the blood in your body concentrates on digestion only. Wait at least 10 minutes, and then walk around for 10 minutes. Or, instead of walking, do the dishes; it should take at least 20 minutes. Once you are done with them, you will see that you are not feeling so full anymore. Or, tell jokes and laugh after the meal to kick-start digestion.

If you overate at a buffet, instead of beating yourself up, complaining, or thinking negatively with feelings of guilt and sadness, get up, go for a walk or go dancing. Thank the Lord for the delicious meal you had. Feel grateful that you are lucky to be eating good food that has variety; it has replenished your system with what was missing. You will immediately start feeling better. Think of how much you enjoyed this meal, forget about what you ate, and focus on the next task at hand—for example, a meeting or a drive—and move on. You can plan to skip the next meal if you are not hungry later on.

Summary: Overate?

- Urinate to make space in your belly
- Do the dishes
- Clean up the living room
- Take a short soft walk
- Crack jokes
- Dance
- Sit there and breathe deeply
- Have a digestive drink (Espresso, White Coffee)
- Do a brain activity, such as reading, writing, or surfing the Internet
- Chew gum (Your system is fooled and expects food so it creates more digestive juices. Do not chew gum for too long because it is not good for your teeth)

You will spark up your system to start burning the energy from the food and get over the fact that you ate too much.

**Eat Late Rarely**
If your body is used to receiving food at night, this is merely a habit and can be relearned. It does not matter what culture you are from, eating past 10 or 11 p.m. is mostly a no-no.

Eat late only when you know you have a long night of studying, working, dancing or travel.

## Never Let a Habit Take Control of You
A princess from the royal family of Abu Dhabi, UAE, once told my mother something, and I found it to be very wise. She said, "I do not like to be controlled by a habit, so I do not let anything *become* a habit."

She was talking about espresso. She had bought a new coffee machine, which made delicious espresso, and when she started feeling like having it too often, she stopped drinking it entirely for a period of time.

## Learn to Say "No" Gently to Yourself and Others
When you are invited to someone's house for a meal, he or she might insist on you eating more of something. If you really want to, okay, but if not, then say, "No, thank you. I am full," politely. Explain yourself. Your choice should not offend anyone's culture. Never eat to please others.

Even if your wife spent all day in the kitchen preparing a meal and you are not hungry because you had too much in the previous meal, say you cannot eat now nicely without upsetting her, but do not eat just to please her; instead, keep her company while she eats.

# Get Out of Obesity

*The only way out is through.*

—Anonymous

Being obsessed with the pleasure of eating, is to an extent a normal thing in humanity, so please do not think that you are sick or that you have a *disorder* (I dislike this word since nothing is permanent). You are no different from someone who obsesses about other pleasures in life such as money, sex, power, drugs, cigarettes or anything that can turn from pleasure to habit, and later on to addiction. The difference is that your challenge is instantly visible when you interact with others, and believe me, there are people out there with worse problems that you cannot see. We are all on this earth to experience life and learn lessons from our mistakes. Enjoy your journey of overcoming your weaknesses, and do not be ashamed that you also have something to work on, just like everybody else.

Assuming that you are eating out of love for food, believe me when I say that the only way to enjoy food to its maximum is by being hungry for it. When you eat it, stop when you are full so that you miss this flavor. Decide to never be driven by your hunger, be conscious when you approach food. Overeating a certain flavor that you adore will diminish your love for it. What you can also do to strengthen yourself when it comes to food is shift your paradigm from quantity to quality. Good quality food makes you feel satisfied and full.

If you are eating due to oversensitivity, then it is no longer about enjoying a nice taste, because constantly eating *diminishes* the pleasure of eating.

On several occasions, please observe yourself when you are in this state of mind and overeating. What are you thinking exactly? When does it happen to you? Is it after an argument with someone? Are you thinking in your mind, *I don't care!* Because you *do* care. If you do not care about yourself, then that could be where this is all coming from.

Once you know what is causing this behavior, it will be easier to figure out a way to stop by asking yourself for help. No one in the world can help you more than you can. You are with yourself all the time, watching every move you make. You cannot hire a dietician to be with you 24 hours a day. You are your own savior. Do not blame it on medication or past events. *Now* is the time you can make a change.

You must not take things out on yourself or others; the battle is out there, not inside you. This will only make you weaker instead of helping you survive your challenges. Life is tough. Accept that, and toughen up so that it will feel normal to you. Monitor yourself over a long period of time; observe and learn more about your own habits. The more you know yourself, the better you can adapt and manage the new lifestyle. Avoid the situations, thoughts, or people that trigger overeating in you, even if they are members of your own family. You know how you got into these habits, and you know that it does not feel good to live like that, so make a change. Start with "the man in the mirror," as Michael Jackson once sang, and get out of there. Start changing your thinking toward yourself; love yourself for who you are, just like God loves us unconditionally. Use your willpower to change; that is why you were given this wonderful trait. Willpower is like a muscle; the more you train it, the stronger it becomes. Patience is a virtue; use it to wait between meals. The most important thing is accepting the shift from being the old you to the new you. Keep this truth in mind: fat melts away, just like you melt butter on a stove. Visualize yourself shrinking and shrinking until your body size becomes what is comfortable for you; even if it takes you two to five years, that is better than having a fast solution that will only take you deeper later. Go for the lifetime change. Do not blame others for making bad food, or cigarettes, etc., because they are unethical and cannot be stopped, forget them and get strong on the inside. You have to fight whatever comes your way.

The fat that is now sitting on your bones in your body remains there, why? Because the new food you are eating these days is sufficient to keep you going on a daily basis in terms of energy for life, so you are burning exactly what you are eating, and all the extra fat in your body is not melting away because you are not programming for that to happen. In order to rid your body of the extra fat, burn much more than you eat. The good news is you have so much energy inside you and you can achieve anything you put your mind to now.

Your main initial focus must be on how to shrink your stomach back to a normal size. Start by avoiding getting full until it hurts. Even if you must eat small meals every three hours instead of one big one that expands your stomach, do that until your stomach shrinks. Amazingly, if you keep your stomach at a reasonable size, you will not feel hungry all the time.

*Do you know what the difference between you and me is?* You walk around carrying 40 or 50 kilos (88 to 110 pounds) more than I do. Imagine yourself thin, but carrying bags weighing around 40 to 50 kilos. It must be really exhausting. When we go shopping, we sometimes want someone to help us carry the bags back home, and those are barely 20 kilos (44 pounds). You are doing this 24 hours a day. The other difference between us is that you are way stronger than I am, and this happens to be the bright side of your situation. The power in your body must be 50 times greater than in mine, because you are so used to handling this weight daily. It means that if you exercise your body, it will immediately develop strong muscles. Train this power within you, and you will be able to apply it to almost anything in life.

If you decide to take the weight off, keep this book with you at all times. Learn all the thoughts in it and the reasoning behind them, and then adapt them to suit your own lifestyle. If you start thinking like me and behaving like me in terms of food habits, you will end up looking great, only stronger ☺. From there on, you will develop habits that suit your lifestyle.

*Hint: I do not want you to want to be me or anyone else; I want you to want to be you.*

118

You might be someone living in Alaska or someone who works late shifts and never sees the sun, so I cannot give you a schedule; you need to figure out your own path. This book will help you keep the weight off once you have reached your goal and have gone on a diet you might have preferred following. You will have to adapt to these great new eating habits and a whole new lifestyle.

Start with the following:

- Love yourself just the way you are.
- Do not bully yourself.
- Be good to you.
- Be your own best friend.
- Give yourself time.
- Forgive the past.
- Forget the past.
- Visualize the new you.

I apologize if I seemed tough in this passage, but sometimes, tough love works better. If you are reading this book, I am assuming that you want to change your life, whereas some people are genuinely happy with their bodies just the way they are.

# Cooking

### Cooking May Be Healthier than Eating at Restaurants
When you make meals at home, you know exactly what is in them. Do not always trust restaurants; they will put anything in food for a good taste. You do not know if they are using canned or expired ingredients or how much oil or butter was used. However, if you do go out occasionally, do not think of what is in the food, and do not feel guilty. Social

eating is a nice activity because you tend to eat more slowly and chew better when surrounded by friends or colleagues, and you end up really enjoying your food.

## Learn to Cook

The ability to cook is a survival tool and will always be an asset to you. The art of cooking is really a wonderful one, and some of the best chefs in the world are men, so being a man is not an excuse. If there is someone in your life doing the cooking for you, such as a wife or mother, then you are lucky, but if I were you, I would ask that person to teach me how to cook and I would occasionally make the dinner myself to get the hang of it.

The best recipes you will find are the ones you get from friends and family, though sometimes you may get lucky and stumble on a nice recipe from the Internet. You will find that the more you enjoy cooking, the better the food.

The Internet is full of recipes; think of your favorite restaurant and the meal you like to order there, and then look it up online to find a good method for cooking it. Whenever you try a recipe that you like, save it in a file on your computer. You can make files by type or country, for example: sweet, savory, American, Middle Eastern, French, and so on.

When you decide to start cooking at home, there will be times when you do not know what to make. Try this: look at what you have as ingredients in the kitchen, and then enter those words in a search engine's box along with the word *recipe*. You are bound to find a recipe that combines those ingredients; you could discover something new. Click on "images" to get many photos of what you are trying to cook. Click on the photo that appeals to you, and most times there will be a recipe on how to make it.

Lots of recipes have too much butter or sugar, so instead of avoiding them entirely, change the recipe to your liking. You have to let yourself long for that little bit of sugar taste instead of overdosing on it. Sometimes less is more.

The same goes for salt, adding too much of it takes away from the natural flavors of the ingredients.

If you are new to cooking, expect the occasional mistakes in the kitchen, such as something not working out, adding the wrong ingredient, or anything else that could happen. I still go through that and learn new things each day. With time, you become much faster and more confident; just be patient with yourself while you learn. Most importantly, try to cook dishes that you have tasted in the past.

*Tip from my sister Rouba: Look at several recipes online of the same dish, and then make your own one.*

### The Do's and Don'ts of Cooking
Remember the danger there is in serving people food that might make them feel sick.

Learn from people who have knowledge and experience, or read about it as much as possible, as there are certain rules in the kitchen that must be memorized. I have gathered a few in this list below:

- To defrost frozen meat, chicken, or fish, let it sit out for a maximum of two hours in summer and then place it in the fridge and let it defrost there. Do not refreeze it after it has been defrosted, even if you cooked it. Also, once defrosted, you must use it within a maximum of two days for meat and chicken and one day for fish, and during those days, it has to be refrigerated.

- Avoid cooking burgers and steaks medium or rare if they were not fresh, and even if fresh, make sure you bought them from a trusted source.

- Fish, if not sushi, must be well cooked, but remember that it cooks quickly and gets dry, with experience you will learn not to over or undercook it.

- Constantly check the expiration date on your goods. Serving dairy products, such as cheese and milk that have expired can immediately make people sick.

- While washing vegetables, rub them well with your fingers and make sure there are no worms or bugs.

- A cut onion gathers bacteria even if you have stored it in the fridge with plastic wrap, so for fresh salads use an onion as soon as you cut it, unless you are planning to fry it with a meal.

- Do an Internet search for the "do's and don'ts of grilling," and for the "do's and don'ts of cooking," you will find lots of useful information there.

- Wooden cutting boards and wooden spoons are contaminated with bacteria, avoid using them, but if you have no choice, then avoid placing raw meat or chicken on them for too long.

### Cooking Is Chemistry, Physics, Math, and Art!
My favorite subject in high school was math, followed by chemistry. I felt bad that I did not make use of these passions during my life, until I realized recently that cooking is chemistry, physics, and math. Cooking is also a form of art, and food itself is chemistry. Knowing this makes cooking so much more interesting because you are stimulating your brain, so do not feel shy if you love it.

### Dinner Party Itinerary Sample
Suppose today is Tuesday and you decide to invite your friends over for a home-cooked meal on Wednesday at 8:00 p.m. (You cannot invite them today because there is not enough time to get ready.) If 8:00 p.m. is dinnertime,

you will need to work your way backward from the time your friends ring the doorbell.

Eating time will be at least 45 minutes from the time people arrive. Some will be late, and others will want to have a chat or a drink before dinner.

*Tuesday 1:00 p.m.:* It is now your lunchtime at work, finish eating and decide on the menu for tomorrow night. Suppose you decide on celery and carrot dips, nuts, spaghetti Bolognese, goat cheese salad, chocolate cake, and drinks. Do not cook a dish for the first time; cook something you know you can make well.

Find out what ingredients you require, and write them down. Figure out what is missing from your kitchen, and plan to go to the supermarket after work on Tuesday, not Wednesday, the day of the dinner.

*Tuesday 7:00 p.m.:* At the supermarket, focus on the things that you need. Do not go into supermarket aisles that do not contain what you require for your dinner. If you plan to bake the cake yourself, it is better to prepare it the night before the dinner unless it is a weekend and you have all day to prepare. If your place needs cleaning, you'd better finish that on Tuesday night as well.

*Wednesday 5:30 p.m.:* You arrive home and start your preparations and cooking. Two and a half hours is good enough to finish up this meal. Chop the celery and carrots first, cook the spaghetti sauce, prepare the salad dressing, followed by the spaghetti and the salad; that way, those last two are fresh for dinnertime. Get dressed and greet your guests. The table can be prepared while your friends are there—sometimes, they enjoy helping you out—unless you had time or prefer to do it by yourself before they arrive. By 8:45 p.m., everything is ready, everybody is hungry, and you can now serve your guests. Right before you serve the salad, turn on the stove to heat the spaghetti sauce. Serve the meals on nice plates and enjoy!

**Cook Healthily**

A lot of the effort in cooking healthily will depend on your logic. Use olive oil instead of most other oils, and do not let it heat up too much before cooking. Decrease the amount of oil you use to the minimum necessary. If you see oil in your dish while eating it, then you must have put in too much of it. Make sure that the person who cooks for you is also health conscious. In general, choose grilled, roasted or steamed instead of deep-fried food. It is amazing what you can do with vegetables and salads. Salads are tasty when the dressing is tasty; otherwise, they can be boring, so get creative with dressings. Get recipes from the Internet, or create them according to your liking. Putting a little sugar or honey in your dressing is okay because at least you are having a salad at the end of the day.

Lightly steam vegetables, and have them with a tasty sauce. You can also refrigerate vegetables you have steamed, and oven-bake them with a nice sauce the following day.

Chop eggplants and potatoes into circles, and zucchini into long strips, brush them with oil and grill them on your electric sandwich maker. When ready, add salt, pepper, and a little olive oil. Make fruit salads, and get creative with them by adding avocados. Invest in a fresh juice maker, and make your own carrot, apple, or celery juices. Avoid having these things every single day so you do not get bored with the taste. Eat protein-filled soybeans, quinoa, or drink soymilk, almond milk, cashew milk or Brazilian nut milk. Regular milk and yogurt contain animal proteins and are also good for you.

In general, live on the lighter side of life!

There are some easy and delicious recipes in *Appendix 1*.

## Work as a Team

Make a system in your home, so you will always be able to cook healthy meals. When you cook, make a lot of everything, so you can eat throughout the week. I find that leftovers taste as good up to five days after having cooked a meal.

If you have a partner, rely on each other and work as a team. Try to get your partner involved in cooking; it is so much more fun to work together in the kitchen and a lot less tiresome. Encourage your partner and congratulate him/her when he/she has created a good meal that you enjoyed. Your diet can have meals from restaurants, but you must have healthy ones that are cooked at home as well.

Learn to cook and compete with your partner on who makes nicer meals. Each one of you might be good at something different.

If you are too hungry to wait for a home-cooked meal, eat, and then cook for the next meal. At home, you mainly cook gourmet food; this is because the ingredients you use are the best and are fresh, not canned. Take a home-cooked meal to work.

If you live on your own, make the effort to cook even if for one person, and occasionally invite a friend or more to indulge with you.

*Tip: The secret to eating healthy is experimenting in the kitchen with healthy ingredients to develop your pallet so that you learn how to make your food taste better.*

## Meal Schedule

The most perfect meal schedule is three medium sized meals a day, with five-hour intervals in between them, and where dinner coincides at 7 p.m.

Shop once a week or every 10 days so that the food is always fresh in your home, and buy everything you feel like eating for that week. Day by day, ask your partner what he or she feels like eating or decide what you feel like eating and cook accordingly. Do not go for food programs that take away the creative part of thinking about what to eat. Your appetite changes and is not like anyone else's. Sometimes, you feel like red meat or quinoa; it all depends on your mood and life circumstances. Besides, food is mood.

# Information

### Read about Food
If you read that natural peanut butter is better for you than peanut butter that has additives and preservatives, then go with the healthier option, especially when both kinds taste the same.

For example, when it comes to calories in food, do not obsess about it by calculating each and every meal you eat. Instead, get a general idea about which foods have lots of calories, and those that do not. You can find all this information on the Internet or buy a small dictionary-type booklet that has the calorie amounts of most kinds of food. Knowing what is heavy and what is light helps you in following the formula: *burn more than you eat*.

### Minimize the Use of the Microwave
An experiment[8] was once conducted to test microwaves. Water was heated in the microwave and then cooled and poured onto the soil of a particular plant; meanwhile, regular boiled water was heated and cooled and was poured onto another plant of the same kind. After a week, the plant that absorbed the water that was microwaved died.

---

8 The Granddaughter of Marshall Dudley conducted this science fair project in 2006 www.execonn.com/sf/

The main reason you should reheat food on a stove is because it becomes brand new again and heats up evenly. It is very simple to do. Put the cold food in a frying pan, and add a little water, or as much as needed, cover the pan and lower the heat. Mix if needed, and after at least 10 minutes, you will get a like-brand-new meal. I lived this way for five years because I do not like microwaves and I am never in a rush to eat.

**Healthy Parents, Healthy Kids**

My parents were unhealthy eaters in their youth until they reached a point in their lives when they just wanted healthy and tasty food to complement their active lifestyle. They served healthy food to their friends and to us, and the response was always positive. We have acquired those good habits at a young age and I am forever grateful.

If your parents did not teach you about healthy food like mine did, then teach yourself; that way, your kids will take it on from you. You may say, my kids dislike healthy snacks or foods, but kids can sometimes be outsmarted. For example, take them to the beach, and let them get really tired and hungry from swimming and playing; when they approach you for a snack, tell them: "Oh no, I forgot the cookies at home! Sorry I only brought these apples and oranges." They will devour them so fast and might change their mind about fruits.

Try other methods to develop your kids' palettes and make them accustomed to healthy food; you know your kids better than I. Remember that these habits will last them a lifetime.

**Benefits of Being Vegetarian**

I lived as a vegetarian for a total of six years. Even though I have not been one for a while, there were many positive benefits I discovered, and I must share them with you:

- Less hair on my legs, as a result of eating less meat from hormone-infused animals.
- Cleaner and healthier teeth.
- More energy to last during the day.
- No more wanting to sleep after lunch.
- No colds, flu, or sore throats.
- No feeling of hunger even after the food in my stomach had been digested.
- No more eating negative energy, the result of the pain and death of an animal; most of the food we eat in restaurants is made from dead cows and chickens frozen from months back. So you could be eating something that has been dead for six months or more.
- I felt lighter, more peaceful, and more positive as a person, as there were no more toxic elements in my system.
- If I felt that I had gained a little weight, I would lose it very fast compared to when I was not vegetarian.

When you have healthy vegetarian meals, you can overeat with no worries.

**Downside of Being Vegetarian**
- I struggled to find tasty vegetarian food because most restaurants do not consider vegetarian people, so their menus contain mostly meat-based meals.
- Mediterranean food was very good because we have plenty of vegetarian starters, but I got bored with it after a while.

If you do not want to turn 100 percent vegetarian, at least do not ask for it in each and every meal.

**Sugar and Salt Levels Can Be Changed**
As you may already know, sugar and salt are a habit. If your level of sugar has gone up tremendously and you now need

to put five teaspoons of sugar into your tea, start bringing it down slowly. To do that, the next time you drink tea or coffee, put one teaspoonful of sugar less than usual, the next time after that, put two teaspoons less, and so on— until the level is normal, like one teaspoon with coffee and two with tea. Another way to bring down your sugar level is to quit cold turkey; drink your coffee or tea without any sugar a few times. Later, you can go back to putting one teaspoon of sugar and you will feel very satisfied by the level of sweetness.

As for salt, always taste your meal before deciding whether it requires more salt. If you feel you are using more salt than other people around you, then it is time to start sprinkling less and less until you do not require much of it. And trust me, this is a habit; once you add too much salt, you will always want that level, unless you bring it down. Then you will be equally happy with less. That way, you can appreciate the natural taste of things.

Additionally, if you make your meals slightly spicy, this adds flavor without the need for extra salt. Spices are beneficial to your blood flow, give you energy, and decrease the chances of heart diseases. To learn to eat spices, you need to bring up your tolerance for spicy chili. One of the reasons people from India are able to stay slim is their use of spices in food which add a lot of flavor without adding a lot of calories.

*Tip:* *The quickest way to bring up your tolerance level to spicy chili is by putting a lot of Tabasco or anything spicy with your next meal, let your mouth burn and your eyes tear, and then do this once or twice more. After that, you will find that the next time you add a reasonable amount of Tabasco to your meal, it will not feel spicy to you.*

## Fake Sugar Keeps You Wanting High-Sugar Desserts

When you eat fake sugar, you are keeping the level of sugar taste in your mouth very high. This is not ideal because you will always seek to reach that level of sweetness by eating high-sugar desserts. Fake sugar drinks are too sweet. One pill of fake sugar equals three teaspoons of regular sugar in taste.

I believe that eating normal sugar is better because the sugar will give you extra energy to work out or burn other things you have eaten and can help digestion. Raw and brown sugar are better than white sugar.

I never touch fake sugar, diet drinks, or diet sweets because they contain chemicals that my body does not recognize, and therefore cannot breakdown. It is a known fact that sugar is not very good for the health either, especially the way it is being produced nowadays; however, few people are able to stop having it altogether, so moderation is important here.

I always wondered why there are no medium-sugar drinks; drinks are always full of sugar or fake sugar. Ready-made coffees, teas, and juices should all have a lower sugar content option.

## How to Handle Your Hunger Before Attacking a Meal

If you are driving your car really fast and you know that soon a traffic light will appear, you do not slam the brakes on suddenly and hurt your car. You gradually slow down, from one gear to the next, until your car comes to a complete stop. Imagine that the traffic light is the meal, and your speed is your level of hunger.

Before you jump into the meal, have a few of these snacks or drinks to diminish your hunger so that when you start the main meal, you will not overeat or eat too fast:

- Water (not optional)
- Carrots

- Apples
- Juices or soft drinks
- Coffee
- Potato chips (with plain yogurt as a dip to balance)
- Baked vegetable chips
- Nuts (preferably raw)
- Beer

## Five-Star, Regular, and Junk-Food Restaurants Compared

The main reason five-star restaurants are expensive is because they use fresh and exotic ingredients, which cost more. In turn, they charge you more, but at least you get better-quality food. The super-talented chef uses creativity for great taste with fewer calories and less oil.

On the other extreme, junk food is heavy with few nutrients or vitamins; it is cheap, and everything in there has been frozen at least six months, though some restaurants are an exception because they use fresh meat, and others grill their meat. The French fries have lots of salt on them, and everything is dipped in fat not oil.

Excess junk food blocks your veins with cholesterol; it is difficult to digest, and it increases cellulite and stretch marks on the body. Unhealthy meals will also leave you feeling drained of energy. I could go on and on about this, but surely health centers have better explanations as to why we should not eat junk food repeatedly. Look at our streets; there are so many fast-food outlets nowadays, and the reason they are there is because we still go and eat the food no matter what health organizations tell us about it, and so do our kids. Those restaurants are there because of our demand for them; they were born out of a necessity to cope with the speed of today's life.

There is a way to enjoy fast food from time to time without doing damage to your body. First we must appreciate that fast-food outlets have made an effort to get healthier by grilling their food instead of frying it, adding low-calorie meals, and adding salads and juices to their menu. I wish they would use real potatoes, change the fat they fry in to a healthier type of oil, and use organic bread for their sandwiches.

Secondly, we must understand exactly what junk food is all about. One, it is about a tasty meal, and two, it is about a fast meal, which makes it convenient during busy times. Do not expect high energy levels in your body after eating it, and do not expect your kids to grow up very strong if they live on it. Let us sum up the junk food don'ts:

- Do not eat it repeatedly or daily.
- Do not let your kids nag you for it; make it a "treat" for them, or just allow it on weekends or at events.
- Avoid it during extremely hot weather because it can cause dehydration.
- Avoid it when you have large work tasks and need lots of energy mentally and physically (unless you are pressed for time), and avoid it on exercise days.

The do's:

- Fast-food meals should not exceed 10 percent of your food intake on a monthly basis.
- Balance it with a healthy and moist meal.
- Have it when you are pressed for time, but eat slowly.
- Have it rarely.
- Look for the outlets that grill their meat.
- Buy a salad with the meal, and share all of the food with someone.
- Drink lots of room-temperature water before eating, and then drink plenty of water one hour after you finish the meal.
- It is better to eat junk food for breakfast or lunch, and the next day eat fruits, vegetables, and beans to dampen your system and regain your energy.
- Make sure you are exercising twice a week to help you digest and burn energy.

This list should keep you safe. Or you can occasionally cook your own fast food at home. I have included the recipe for homemade burgers in *Appendix 1*. At least you are having fresh minced meat and you know how much fat is in it. French fries made at home from fresh potatoes are yummy, so have them occasionally.

Some non-five stars, non-fast food restaurants also use fresh ingredients, so their food is healthy and tasty, but high in calories. The calories in some regular chicken dishes at restaurants can range from 1,200 to 1,600 calories in one dish. You are better off ordering one main meal and one salad and sharing both those with a friend, or taking some home, unless you are very hungry and your body needs those calories.

If you have no choice but to eat out, then find healthy places to go to or make the effort to pick up ready-made meals from a well-reputed food market.

*Survey Results for Restaurant Choice*

**Most Visited Restaurants**

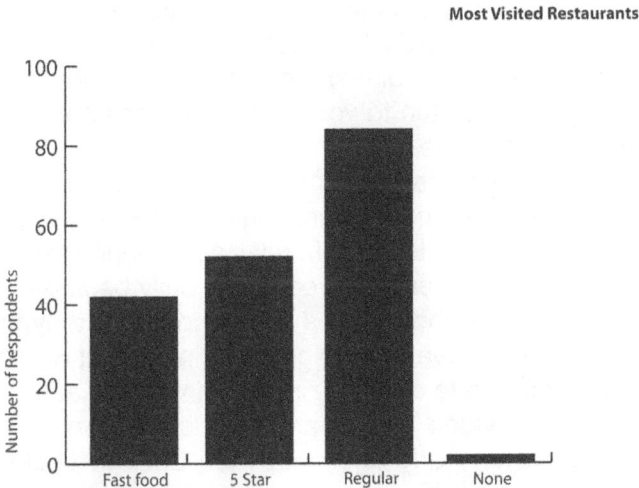

133

## Skip Meals When Required, Not Daily

A person feels less hungry while he or she is in action mode, hungrier while doing minimal activity, and lazy when too full. Therefore, a person ought to focus more on consuming the energy in food, rather than eating.

As mentioned earlier, the idea behind skipping meals is to ensure that you eat when your body needs it and when you are hungry; this way, you will avoid piling up energy in your system that is not going to be used in the near future, and you will enjoy the taste better.

I do not encourage skipping the same meal daily, because you are improvising with food; you need that meal sometimes to balance yourself.

Suppose that, on your weekend, you decide to stay home all day and relax watching movies. Since you wake up later than usual on your weekend, and you are not as active as on a working day, there is no need to have three full meals. You can have two or as much as needed because there is no big activity happening that day to require all that energy from food.

If you had a heavy meal late on a particular night, skip breakfast; in other words, burn *before* you eat. If you had a late, heavy lunch, skip dinner, especially if you do not feel hungry at dinner. Listen to your body; if it does not require anything, do not force it.

Sometimes you can skip meals earlier; for example, if you are invited to a dinner where you know there will be lots of food and you want to enjoy it, have a light lunch that day.

Children need to eat all three meals daily because they are still developing their bodies and minds, until they have passed 21. If you have overweight kids, instead of worrying about it, concentrate on engaging them with fun activities, away from the video games and television. They should understand at an early age, that food and fat could be burned with activities.

Make sure your eating time coincides with others, so that you are not left out eating at an odd hour and alone. This will be perfected with practice.

Start by asking yourself or reviewing what you ate before. Answer honestly whether you think your body needs another meal or snack, and trust your logic. For example, if you are going on a long driving trip, you need energy to stay awake, so do not choose to skip a meal before that.

Take each situation as it comes, so when you want to have the next meal, that is when you think of what you will eat depending on how hungry you are, what the event is, what texture is important next, what you last ate, and what is happening next in your schedule. Your meals must contain vitamins and nutrients to keep you energized at all times.

You can overeat occasionally, like when the food is unbelievably amazing or you are at a buffet or event, but not just for the sake of it.

Do not have too many consecutive meals that are heavy, with the hope of balancing them out later. Now is when you need to balance, so do not pile up work for later; work on it now.

Whenever you skip any meal, have lots of water during those hours.

Healthy meals give you energy to burn everything that enters your body; so do not skip meals if you have had a series of unhealthy meals because you will feel weak. I know you are trying to burn calories, but that is not the way.

During a stressful time at work, if you have had no breakfast and no lunch, be careful; you might be hungrier than you think, so force yourself to eat so that you do not faint. Sometimes we are so stressed at work and this causes our stomachs to shrink and we do not feel hungry when in fact we need a lot of energy from food.

*Note: since you are not counting calories, your best indicators to know when and what to eat next are your logic and hunger level.*

# Movement

It is amazing how people always try to avoid movement. They want to park their car right in front of the place they are going to; they want to take a taxi instead of walking; they would rather buy a car and not rely on public transport because it involves lots of walking; and they take the elevator instead of the stairs. On the contrary! Move! If you have no time to walk then leave earlier.

Unless you are a builder or something like that, work today involves mostly sitting at a desk. That burns calories, but not enough. Try to move about any chance you have. If you forgot something in the car that you require now, get up and get it, and do these nice things for others.

At the office, go and do the photocopying instead of asking the office assistant. Moving about keeps your blood flowing at a reasonable pace and aids digestion. If you do not move enough during the day, your metabolism slows down.

My husband leaves his car at home several days in a week, and walks to work.

*Tip: A weekend spent out in the sun hiking or in the park is much better than one spent sitting on the couch. It will leave you feeling more energized and ready to face a new working week.*

## Keep Active at Any Age

If you are over 60 years of age and find that your days are quite empty, take on a new challenge. Thomas Jefferson started building the University of Virginia at age 82. Your spirit's desire to work, learn and have fun never ages, so live young and keep active.

My wonderful mother-in-law, a school nurse, has a great body. She is so beautiful and looks 20 years younger than her age. I once asked her what her secret is, and she said, "I always take the stairs." What she meant was that in any given situation where there is a choice of easy versus difficult, she always chooses the difficult way, the one that involves more work (i.e. the stairs).

While living with her for a while, I observed her eating habits and found that she does not deny herself the things she likes. If she is not at work, she is up on her feet and doing something in the house.

Her life revolves around her grandchildren, God bless them, and so she creates many activities with them. She also organizes events for her family, sends lovely cards and gifts to all her loved ones, meets friends, invites people over for dinner, goes out to play bridge or whatever she and her husband like to do, cycling, swimming, and walking. She spends the entire year working hard for her community. She is a giver, and that requires a lot of energy, hence the great body she has.

I asked my father-in-law, who is a general practitioner, the same question about the secret to his great body and health at his age. His answer was that in addition to doing some of the activities his wife does, he runs his own medical clinic, repairs his cars and appliances at home in his workshop, eats dinner early, and still finds time to do 30 minutes of stretching for his back muscles and 30 minutes of exercise per day, five times a week; he too takes the stairs and parks his car far from the entrance to his destination.

This is something my husband does too; I could not understand the logic behind it until he explained it to me. Basically, at a busy shopping center or department store, it is easier and faster to park far away from the entrance. It is often busy near the entrance, since everyone else is trying to park there, so it takes longer to find a parking spot, and if you do manage to find one, it takes longer to get out of the spot after shopping because of all the cars trying to park near the entrance. By parking farther away, you get more walking done.

**Use All Your Senses**
Taste and smell are two senses that are used intensely during eating. Why do you keep stimulating the same two senses? There are other senses you can stimulate to feel happy and alive. If you find yourself eating out of boredom, stop and find something to stimulate your other senses, the ones that consume energy. Try combining them in different ways.

Here are some ways you can stimulate your senses:

- Touch—Hold your kids, spouse, or family member. Touch the sand on the beach. Have a massage. Create art.
- Sight—Take photos in nature. Go to the beautiful, magical desert or to a mountain. Watch your kids playing. Go see a movie. Visit an art gallery, museum, or park. Read a book. Start a blog. Surf the Internet. Go for a drive and enjoy nice scenery, or walk on the marina. *Note: Avoid watching television, it drains you of energy.*
- Sound—Listen to music. Listen to your kids singing.
- Smell—Smell flowers or visit a candle or soap shop.
- Sight and sound—Walk on the beach, see and hear the ocean waves hit the shore. Watch a musical play.
- Sight and taste—Invite friends for tea and scones, visit a vineyard.
- All senses—Visit a new country.

Live your life. Do not spend it sitting and waiting; use your time creatively. Revolve around the beauty and richness of life and not just around eating. There is so much to do and not everything requires money. Be creative and spontaneous, not every activity requires lots of planning.

*Tip: Close your eyes while eating, your sense of taste will magnify.*

## In Cold Weather, You Burn More Energy
In cold weather, do not keep your heat switched on the entire day and night; this will make you feel lethargic. The best time to switch on the heating is for a couple of hours in the morning when you get out of bed, and for another two hours around sunset. During the night, use warm covers and turn off the heat, unless of course you live in a place where the temperature is way below freezing.

During all the other hours of the day, leave a small crack in the window to get some fresh air to keep you energetic and lively. If you are active around the house or outside, your body will use up energy to warm itself up. Call a friend. Avoid just sitting down in one place. Keep moving.

## Stay Active during and after Pregnancy
I do not have children, so I gathered advice from what I have heard over the years and also from a few ladies who have been pregnant and were kind enough to share their experience and learning with the world.

Stay fit during your pregnancy; being pregnant should not be an excuse for you to sit down and do nothing. This way, your child will be much healthier at birth, your delivery will be smoother, and your confidence and morale will be higher. Of course, you need to do a very gentle workout. Swimming, walking, and yoga for pregnant women are perfect.

Drinking water gradually and slowly is very important during pregnancy.

Women who have just given birth need to become more active; with a newborn it will just happen anyhow. Take the baby out for walks and fresh air. Take up swimming or a new sport. Take your time; losing the weight can take at least six months to a year. Do not worry it is only fat, figuratively speaking, it melts like butter on a stove. Thank God extra weight is not actually made of iron!

It is easier and more effective to keep in shape during pregnancy than to lose a big chunk at the end of it.

You do not have to gain so much weight and use pregnancy as an excuse to binge. Unlike common belief, you do not have to eat for two people. Eat healthy, and minimize junk food and meat.

I was amazed while reading one of the questionnaires when an Indian woman claimed she could not eat meat during her pregnancy; she became a vegetarian until after she gave birth. It happened naturally.

Be careful what you eat because it impacts the child directly, so think twice about what you consume and avoid the obvious—alcohol, coffee/caffeine products, pills, and raw seafood—while pregnant and while breastfeeding. Drink lots of herbal teas.

Most women claimed their appetite and hunger levels grew at the beginning of the pregnancy but then adjusted back to normal toward the middle and end. If you are used to eating large portions as a new habit, it is better to eat vegetarian food for a while, because you can eat double the portion and your body will dispose of it quickly. Breastfeeding helps you to lose weight too, because your body needs lots of energy to produce new milk.

Use this book to get back into shape after giving birth; a lot of the things here do not apply to you while you are pregnant or breastfeeding, especially skipping meals or doing certain types of exercise like hiking because it can be dangerous.

## Sunbathing Followed by Swimming

The sun is good for you; it helps your body make Vitamin D.

Assuming that you like being tanned, a great way to shape your body fast is in the summer and can be done while sunbathing followed by swimming.

At the beach or pool, apply sun block cream on your face and body, or oil with protection on your body if your skin can handle it. Spend equal time (20 minutes) on your front side and back side. While you are lying there, keep putting water on your head, or else you risk sunstroke. After 40 minutes, jump in the pool or ocean and swim around. Do not just float there, or it is a wasted opportunity to burn energy. Then do it again: tan for 40 minutes (20 minutes on each side) and then swim a lot, at least 15 to 30 minutes; it really helps to be in cold water because your body uses up energy to warm itself up. If the water is cold, it helps to tighten your skin for a great look.

If you do this regularly in the summer, you will have a gorgeous tan and your body will be toned. Take a walk on the beach and burn more calories—my father's favorite activity—remember to wet your hair.

Be very careful of the sun if it is too hot outside. Avoid exposure between the hours of midday and 3:00 p.m., as it would be best to lie in the shade of an umbrella. You really need to use your logic on this one. Remember to use protection and do not lie in the sun for too long.

# Sleep

### Sleep Six to Eight Hours

An active body needs proper rest, and this will aid in weight loss. Your body needs at least seven hours of rest to digest well, recover, and have energy. If you are tired, you will not feel happy and energetic enough to work out and be on top of your life. If you are busy and can only manage a few long nights of sleep a week, then try to balance it out on weekends.

If you cannot sleep the same amount of hours each night, what you can do is improvise—sleep six hours three times a week, nine hours two times a week, eight hours once a week, and twelve hours once a week.

*Tip: in order to get out of bed easily in the morning, avoid using covers that make you very hot during your sleep, medium warmth is healthy.*

## Ways to Fall Asleep

If you cannot fall asleep easily or wake up during the night, here are some ideas to help you:

- Breathe through your nose and actively listen to the breathing you are doing with no other thoughts on your mind.
- Close the thoughts in your mind like you close the browser windows on a computer screen.
- Lights out.
- Read.
- Try meditation while lying in bed, relaxing part by part. Relax your feet, then your calves, followed by your knees, and so on until you relax your eyes, your jaw, and finally your mind. You may be asleep by then.
- Go to the toilet; a full bladder sometimes results in no sleep, or your body might wake you up at night to urinate.
- Drink water; sometimes your body wakes you up during your sleep because it wants more water for digestion. If you do not drink, you may not be able to go back to sleep, so keep a water bottle near your bed every night.
- Work out; it will make you tired enough to fall asleep.

# Remedies for the Body

## Medication Needs Your Healing Powers
When you take medication for an illness, your body is also doing the healing, not just the pill; the pill cannot fix the problem without your genuine belief that you will get better. The problem with drugs is that they make the body dependent on them, so you will need to keep taking pills instead of depending on your own system. (Consult your doctor if you have decided to stop any current medication that was prescribed to you in the past.)

## Shower in the Evening
If you only want to shower once a day, better to do so in the evening after work; that way, you will wash off all the sweat from a hard day's work. You disconnect and enjoy your evening with your family, and then go to sleep clean and positive, since showers really do put you in a good mood. Do not take the dirt to your bed.

Do not shower right before sleep, because you will have a humid body in bed, and this is not healthy. Shower at least one hour before bedtime.

Morning showers are better if you slept late and need to freshen up before work.

## Detoxify on Some Weekends
One of my favorite former roommates used to have what she called a "detox weekend." This was an entire weekend in which she did not drink alcohol or eat heavy meals; everything was liquid. You can have these when you feel that your week was stuffed with heavy lunches or dinners because of business meetings. You can have lots of soups and fresh juices even if only for one day on the weekend every once in a while.

## Sit with Good Posture Especially while Eating

While eating, maintain good posture. If you sit up straight and get close to the table, there will be reasonable space in your belly; you will feel the fullness in time and not overeat. If your neck is slouched forward, pull your head back, and try to imagine that the back of your head is aiming to touch the ceiling.

For good posture, sit on your buttocks not on your spine. When you slouch and place your buttocks at the edge of a chair or sofa, you will end up sitting on the bottom of your spine and not upright, this can hurt your back on the long run.

*Try it now: In your chair sit as far back as possible. Stick out your butt-cheeks and sit on them as if they were pillows, and you will find that your spine is naturally and easily upright.*

## How to Deal with a Hangover

Alcohol in moderation is better than in large quantities in the same night, but if you overdrank alcohol one night, this will most probably turn into a major and painful hangover the following day. To avoid the headache, and only in this case, eat half a cheese sandwich before going to bed. If you forget to do that, then drink plenty of water the next day after breakfast. Also, avoid drinking on an empty stomach or mixing many types of alcohol; stick to one or two types a night.

## The Ocean—A Healing Place

When you go swimming in the ocean, you cleanse your mind, body, and soul. The salt water purifies your body. This helps you deal with stress. The sound of the birds and waves is serene and calming.

Some people are now so afraid of everything, they think the sun gives them cancer and the ocean is dirty. Do not live your life in disgust or fear of what might go wrong; just go out there and live the moment. We are part of everything on this earth. Do not separate yourself.

## Aloe Vera
The Aloe Vera plant has a healing effect on the body. For cuts, burns, or simply younger-looking skin, my parents swear by this stuff. There was a time when they would give out Aloe Vera plants to friends as a gift. To use this plant cut a branch, slice the thorns off, and then slice it in the middle and apply its gel on the area you want to heal or directly on your face as you would apply a facial mask.

## Massages
To relax the body and tone the muscles, have massages once a month. It helps to oxygenate the areas in your muscles that are stiff and that are working the most when you are at the gym.

If you are working out regularly, you will enjoy massages more. Find out which style suits you best, such as Aromatherapy or deep tissue. You can massage yourself but will not be able to reach all areas. You and your partner can take turns.

## Back Pain
Your back can hurt in different areas. Try to figure out what you are doing to yourself on a daily basis that could be causing the pain; either you are sitting in one wrong posture at your desk for too long, sleeping on the wrong mattress, doing harmful movements during exercise, not exercising at all, carrying heavy things during your job while putting the weight on your back instead of your leg muscles, not stretching properly before and after workouts, standing up

for too long at work, doing housework for many hours while hunched over, or many other reasons.

The best remedy for the back is to stretch it regularly, and not only when it hurts, that way, you are ensuring that your muscles are not getting tight, and that the blood is flowing normally.

> *Try this simple stretch: Lie down on the ground on your back, hug your knees tightly with both arms, let the knees touch your chest, drop one leg and keep hugging the other one; switch legs and repeat. Breathe deeply whenever you stretch and take your time.*

Another back stretch is to stand up straight, let your head fall toward your feet while keeping the knees slightly bent, and roll up slowly, vertebra by vertebra, starting from the lower back until you straighten up. Do this at least three times in a row.

The other obvious remedy is swimming; it strengthens your back muscles and coordinates your entire body.

**Teeth**

Rinse your teeth with water after sweets, chocolate, and coffee. Those substances enter in between your teeth and gums and work quickly to decay them. You do not have access to a toothbrush everywhere, so if you sip drinking water and rinse your teeth twice as soon as you finish consuming any of these three, you will keep your teeth safer. You only get one set of teeth as an adult, so treat them right.

Brush your teeth two or three times a day; more is not good for them. Before bedtime, floss after brushing, and then rinse with water. Floss carefully in front of a mirror, be sure to take out the food by flossing and not squash it further up into your gums. Wash the floss thread if it gathers too much food before continuing to floss the remaining teeth.

## Holidays

Detaching yourself from work is healthier than you think. You always come back with new ideas and a rejuvenated mind and body. People who do not know how to enjoy their time off because of budget constraints or fear of losing money are actually wasting this time given to them to relax, disconnect, and de-stress. Once back at work, you will want to reconnect and restart a brand-new year filled with new resolutions and renew your dedication to your work, making money, and living a healthier lifestyle.

## Healing

If you have had serious injuries, heart problems, operations, separations, or any other diagnosis at a hospital or clinic, do not let that stop you from going on. You are capable of healing yourself, and this is something no one can do for you.

While watching the 2012 Olympics, I was amazed by some of the stories that demonstrated willpower and determination. Bryshon Nellum, a runner from Southern California who had been shot four times in both legs back in 2008, had healed from surgery and was competing in the 2012 Olympics. What a story!

## Smile ☺

The face has so many muscles; they are shaped by our thoughts, feelings, and words. The more you think sad, lonely, negative thoughts, the more your face will permanently be shaped by those emotions. Erase the past, and start over. Reshape your face with positive, loving, and happy thoughts. Watch this silent film for inspiration. On YouTube, search for "Beat Wrinkles Naturally" or use this link: http://www.youtube.com/watch?v=UKQhGJsO4uM.

\* \* \*

# CONCLUSION

Figure out your real gifts, because their memory is what will be left behind on earth when you die. No one will remember your weight; they will remember your inner beauty and your contributions to society so create a purpose for your existence and fulfill it.

Love all that you have been given; do not complain about your life, especially your body. Happiness is so simple to attain; just decide to be happy, count your blessings daily, enjoy what you have while you have it because everything is temporary.

Remember, it is not about how you look; it is about how you feel and how you feel in general about yourself, so stay confident!

Close your eyes, and picture the new you:

Awake
Balanced
Connected
Contained
Coordinated
Content
Happy
Positive
Upright
Marvelous

Peaceful
Logical
Conscious
Confident
Centered

Let the light in your healthy heart shine through!

\* \* \*

## Months or Years after You Read *Great Body No Diet*

Okay, so you have lost weight and you feel great. You love how balanced you are. All of a sudden you feel like you are gaining weight so you start panicking. Perhaps what really happened was that you followed the *burn more than you eat* formula for a while but eventually stopped? Relax and know that you will turn things around again, stay strong. Once you decide to get healthy again, that feeling alone will give you the confidence you need to be on top of things, and you will be able to go back to the weight you like. It may help to reread this book.

\* \* \*

If you benefited from and enjoyed reading *Great Body No Diet*, I would love to hear your thoughts so please write a review on Amazon.com, I would really appreciate that.
Do like the book page on Facebook and follow me on Twitter @rachazeidan.

Thank you for reading! God bless you!

# APPENDIX 1

## Cooking Methods and Recipes

Everyone has different recipes for common things—for food, for love, for confidence, and for chemistry. That is what makes us all so special and different.

Learn these simple and yummy recipes and cooking methods to get you started in the habit of cooking.

## Rice

### Basmati Rice or Jasmine Rice
Cook it on high heat like you would cook pasta, with lots of **water,** a pinch of **salt**, and **a** drop of **vegetable oil**, (or cook it as directed on its packaging). After 15 minutes or more, taste the rice to be sure that it is as cooked as you want; if it is, take the pot off the heat, run fresh cold water through it, drain the rice and place it back in the same pot. Cover the pot with aluminum foil and then its cover, and keep it on low heat for 5 minutes.

Basmati rice is light, and its cooking method allows you to wash out the starch that gathers in the water.

### Egyptian Rice with Vermicelli

Cook a quarter of a cup of **vermicelli** with a little bit of **vegetable oil**; keep stirring it and watching it until it turns brown. Add the **Egyptian rice**; for each 1 cup of rice, add 1 ½ cups of **cold water**, and then add a pinch of **salt**. Allow it to cook on low heat covered for 15 to 30 minutes or until the water is completely absorbed.

### Baked Goods

Whenever you buy or make baked goods such as croissants, scones, bread, muffins, or French baguette bread, the best way to preserve them is by freezing them the evening of the first day. When you want to eat them again, put them in the oven for as long as they need to become fresh again.

# Vegetables

*Tip: When you buy fresh vegetables, before you put them in your refrigerator, do not wash them, wrap them with acid-free paper or a newspaper and then place them in their original plastic bag. This will help to absorb the wetness they contain and make them last longer in your fridge.*

*Wash vegetables when you are ready to use them in your meals.*

### Zucchini with Rice (Easy, light, and fast)

Chop 2 cloves of **garlic**, 1 **onion**, and a small piece of **fresh ginger** (optional). Add them to ¼ cup of **pine nuts**, and fry all of these in a pot with some **olive** (preferred) **or vegetable oil** until brown. Chop 4 **zucchinis** into cubes or half circles, and add them to the pot, lightly fry them, and then add 4 to 5 cups of **plain tomato sauce** from a box or glass container. Cook on low for about 20 minutes. Add

**salt, pepper,** and **chili powder** to your liking. Serve with **basmati or jasmine rice**.

### Steamed Vegetables
To make **vegetables** interesting after you have steamed them is by sautéing them in **teriyaki sauce** and adding **herbs, salt,** and **pepper**. Or make a **garlic** and **lemon** sauce or **garlic** and **butter** sauce. You can try this veggie combination: green beans, potatoes, zucchini, and cauliflower. Or this one: potatoes, carrots, Brussels sprouts, and broccoli.

### Garlic Sauce Recipe for Steamed Vegetables
½ garlic **clove**, 1 to 2 tablespoons of **vinegar** (not balsamic), 1 to 2 tablespoons of **lemon juice**, 2 to 3 tablespoons of **olive oil**, and **herbs**. Mix them all together, and serve on warm (not hot) steamed **vegetables**.

### Grilled Vegetables
Chop large rounds of **potatoes**, an **eggplant**, and **zucchini**; brush with **olive oil**, and cook for approximately 20 minutes on your electric grill. Sprinkle with **salt** and **pepper**, and serve as a starter.

### Homemade Fries
Chop fresh **potatoes**; in a pot, heat enough **oil** to sink the chopped potatoes into. Cook on high heat until golden brown. Place them on kitchen paper to absorb the oil and put **salt** on them to your liking. (This meal cooks better on gas stoves as opposed to electric.)

### Mashed Potatoes
Boil or steam **potatoes**. Mash them with a special tool or fork. Heat **milk** and **butter** and add them to the potatoes as desired and then put **salt** and a pinch of **white pepper**.

**Baked Potatoes with Sour Cream and Baked Garlic on the Side**

Bake **potatoes** and an entire **garlic bulb** in the oven by placing them on the bottom rack. Turn them upside down once they become dark brown. Serve with **sour cream**, **cheese**, or your favorite toppings.

# Pasta

**Penne Arabiatta (Serves 4):**

Put 6 tablespoons of **olive oil** in a pot, and add 4 **cloves of garlic**. Cook until light brown, and then add a can of peeled **plum tomatoes or tomato sauce**, a teaspoonful of **tomato paste**, and a cup of hot **water**. Cook for 20 minutes on low to medium heat. Then mash them all together while they are still cooking. Next, add a tablespoon of **milk** and some fresh **basil**, **red chili** powder, **salt**, and **pepper**, and turn the heat off.

Meanwhile, add some **olive oil** and **salt** to a pot filled with hot **water**; cook 250 g of penne until soft (but not too soft). Mix with the tomato sauce, and serve with a pinch of grated **Parmesan cheese** and cracked **black pepper**.

# Meat

**Spaghetti Bolognese**

Fry 1 chopped **onion** with 4 **garlic cloves** and **carrots** (optional) chopped into tiny cubes. Add **pine nuts** (optional), and once browned, add fresh chopped **mushrooms** (optional). In another pot, add a quantity that you like of **mincemeat**. Let it cook for a while. If the mincemeat was frozen, wait for it to thaw, and add 2 tablespoons of **milk** and 2 tablespoons of **white or red wine**. Once the juice has been absorbed, add a teaspoon of **black pepper**.

Then add 2 glass bottles of **tomato sauce**. Add fresh or dry **basil**; let it cook covered for at least 20 minutes stirring occasionally. Once it is ready, add **salt** and **chili** (optional). During the 20-minute wait, prepare the **pasta** by placing it in boiling **water** with a pinch of **salt** and a drop of **olive oil**. Cook it for 10 to 15 minutes or as per instructions on the pack. Once ready, wash off the starch, and then serve it with the sauce and a pinch of grated **Parmesan cheese** and cracked **black pepper**.

### Spinach and Mincemeat with Basmati Rice (Easy, light, and fast. Omit meat for a vegetarian version)

Cook half lb of **mincemeat** or less, with 1 **onion** in **olive oil** until well done; add a handful of **pine nuts**, and cook them until brown.

Add a large quantity of washed **fresh spinach**, half a cup of **water**, and cover. After 10 minutes, the spinach will seem to vanish to nearly ¼ of the original quantity placed in the pot. Mix all the ingredients together, and cook for another 15 minutes, then add a pinch of **salt** and **black pepper** and **chili**. Cook some basmati rice as indicated earlier. Once ready to eat, place spinach on top of the rice in your plate, and sprinkle it with a little bit of fresh **lemon juice**.

### Homemade Burgers

With your clean hands, or using disposable plastic gloves, mix **mincemeat**, 1 **egg**, 1 grated **onion**, **salt**, **pepper**, and ¼ cup of **breadcrumbs**, and then shape into burgers. Or you can omit all those ingredients and just use mincemeat. With a paper towel, lightly grease the frying pan (omit oil if the pan is non-stick) and fry the burger patties to rare or medium, if using fresh meat, and well done if using frozen meat. Or you can place them on a grilling machine instead of frying. Add any of the following toppings such as **lettuce, fresh tomato, fried or fresh onions, ketchup, mayo,**

**mustard, Tabasco or cheese**. Serve with homemade **fries** and a side **salad**.

# Chicken

### Chicken Hotel Kevin
Fry 1 **onion** with 3 **garlic cloves** and a slice of **fresh ginger**, add 2 chopped **carrots**, add 2 or 3 **chicken breasts** cut into cubes. Add 1.5 teaspoons of **turmeric powder**, a pinch of **cayenne powder** and a pinch of **curry powder** (optional). Add ½ a litre of **cream** (double or single) or **coconut milk** (optional) and a bit of **water** as much as you think is right.

Add dry **oregano** and 1 **bay leaf**. After the meal has cooked for 20 minutes, add **salt** and **pepper** to taste, followed by green or yellow **squash** at the end during the last 5 minutes of cook time so that it does not get overcooked and soggy. Serve with **basmati or jasmine rice**.

# Soups

### Carrot
Fry 1 chopped **onion** with **oil**; add 6 chopped **carrots** and 2 chopped **celery** sticks, and fry them together. Add 2 large cups of **water** to a pot, and bring to a boil. Once boiled, let it cool off a little. Blend them, and add **salt**.

### Vegetable
Fry 1 chopped **onion**; add **fresh ginger**. Chop 2 **carrots**, 1 **celery** stalk, and 3 small **zucchini/squash**. Add one **vegetable stock** cube. Add 4 cups of **water** and cook for 20 minutes.

**Pumpkin**

Fry 1 large **onion**. Add 2 chopped **carrots**. Boil in 1 cup of **water**. In the oven, cook chopped **pumpkin** with **oil**. Once pumpkin is ready, add to the carrots and boil. Once boiled, let it cool off a little, and blend them together. Add **salt**. Serve each bowl with a teaspoonful of unsweetened **whipped cream**.

**Red Lentil**

Fry 1 chopped **onion** in your favorite **oil**. Chop 2 **celery** stalks and 2 **carrots**. Add them to the **onions**. Add 5 cups of **water**. Once the vegetables are cooked, add 1 cup of **red lentils** and boil until cooked. Add 1 teaspoon of **salt** and 2 teaspoons of **cumin powder**. Let it cool off a little and blend until smooth. Serve each bowl with a squeeze of **lemon juice** and some dry **pita bread** pieces.

# Salads

There are many possible combinations for salads as follows:

1. Avocado, lettuce, corn, mushrooms, and tomatoes served with lemon and olive oil dressing or balsamic vinegar with olive oil.
2. Rocket leaves (arugula), Parmesan cheese, pine seeds, and pumpkin or cranberries with balsamic vinegar dressing.
3. Walnuts with sun-dried tomatoes, rocket leaves, and a balsamic vinegar dressing.

The range of combinations is endless. Look at restaurant menus or search the Internet for additional ideas.

# Salad Dressings

1. Balsamic vinegar, ½ teaspoon of water, olive oil, and pinch of basil, salt, pepper
2. Lemon, honey, olive oil, basil, salt, and pepper
3. Lemon, finely crushed mint leaves with salt, olive oil
4. Lemon, ½ teaspoon mustard (any type), olive oil, salt, and pepper

Interesting additions to salad dressings include: maple syrup, agave, sugar, honey, jam, yogurt, mayo, mustard, and sour cream.

# Cakes

Cake recipes have to be followed perfectly; you cannot change the recipe except by decreasing sugar to your liking.

Try these yummy recipes that I learned from my friends in New Zealand.

**Banana Cake**
125 g **butter**, softened
¾ cup **sugar**
3 **eggs**
Drop of **vanilla**
1 cup mashed **bananas**
1 teaspoon **baking soda**
2 tablespoons hot **milk**
2 cups plain **flour**
1 teaspoon **baking powder**
1 portion of **Cream Cheese Icing**

Prepare the cake dish by rubbing butter on it, add a pinch of flour so the cake does not stick, and turn the oven on at a temperature of 180°C (350°F).

Mix butter and sugar until light and fluffy. Add eggs one at a time, beating well after each addition. Add mashed bananas, and mix thoroughly. Stir baking soda into hot milk, and add to creamed mixture. Sift flour and baking powder together. Stir into mixture. Add the batter to the cake dish. Bake at 180°C (350°F) for 50 minutes or until cake springs back when lightly touched. Leave in tin for 10 minutes before turning out onto a wire rack. The mixture can also be baked in two 20 cm round sandwich tins at 180°C for 25 minutes.

When cooled, ice with chocolate, lemon, or passion fruit icing or the cream cheese icing that follows.

## Cream Cheese Icing
1 tablespoon **butter**, softened
½ cup **cream cheese**
1 cup **icing sugar**
½ teaspoon grated **lemon rind**

Beat the butter and cream cheese until creamy.
Mix in icing sugar and lemon rind, and beat well to combine.
Spread over cake.

## Chocolate Cake
Prepare the cake dish by rubbing butter on it, add a pinch of flour so the cake does not stick, and turn the oven on at a temperature of 180°C (350°F).

4 oz (100 g) of **Butter**
8 oz (200 g) of **Sugar**
2 tablespoons of **Maple syrup**

Mix all the previous ingredients in a pot over medium heat, by melting the butter and maple syrup first. Sift and add 10 oz of **flour** and 2.5 teaspoons of **baking powder** with 3 tablespoons of **chocolate powder**, mix in a ¼ cup of **orange juice** or less if you feel like it with a drop of **brandy or whisky** (optional) with a drop of **vanilla** and 2 **eggs**, mix well, then add to the hot pot, mix them quickly.

In a small pot, add one cup of **fresh milk**, wait until before boil and that is when you add ½ a teaspoon of **baking soda** and mix well. Add a cube of Bakers **semi-sweet chocolate** (optional) to the cake mixture. Add the milk to the chocolate and mix well, then place the batter in the metal cake dish, and bake for 30 minutes or until cake springs back when touched. Once cooled, slice in middle to add the following chocolate sauce, and cover it with sauce on the outside as well. Serve it with vanilla ice cream. If you eat it the next day, place a slice of cake in the microwave for 20 seconds before serving.

**Chocolate Sauce a la Rouba**
In a small pot and over the stove, heat up 100ml of liquid **whipping cream**. Once it gets hot add 7 oz (200 g) of **semi-sweet chocolate** for cooking, cut into pieces. Mix well until it thickens then spread it inside and over the cake.

\* \* \*

# APPENDIX 2

## Shopping List

Here is a list that you can photocopy and follow each time you go to the supermarket to do your routine shopping; it contains most of the ingredients of every recipe mentioned earlier and more.

- Basmati or jasmine rice, Egyptian white rice, brown rice, noodles
- Olive oil, sunflower oil, butter, apple vinegar, balsamic vinegar, lemon, teriyaki sauce, soy sauce
- Salt, herbs, nutmeg, pepper, seven spices, dry oregano, fresh basil, chili powder, cumin, turmeric, cayenne, sugar, brown sugar, powder sugar
- Pine nuts, walnuts, and almonds (freeze them to make them last longer)
- Garlic, onions, fresh ginger
- Minced meat, chicken, steaks, escalope, seafood
- Carrots, fresh mushrooms, eggplant, green beans, potato, zucchini, cauliflower, potatoes, carrots, Brussels sprouts, broccoli, lettuce, corn, cucumbers, tomatoes, avocado, celery, green salad leaves of all types, fresh mint, carrots, rocket leaves, sun-dried tomatoes, spinach, pumpkin
- Red lentils, brown lentils

- Fruits, including bananas, oranges and watermelon (during the summer) and anything else you like
- White or red wine and beer
- Pasta (spaghetti and penne), vermicelli (for the Egyptian rice), noodles
- Peeled plum tomatoes (in a can), tomato paste, tomato sauce, vegetable stock cubes
- Ketchup, mayo, mustard, Tabasco
- Cheese, cream cheese, eggs, fresh milk, soy milk, organic rice milk, Parmesan cheese, yogurt, fresh cream, whipped cream
- Hamburger buns, pita bread, toast bread, breadcrumbs
- High-fiber cereals
- Coffee, tea
- Honey, maple syrup
- Baking soda, icing sugar, flour, baking powder, chocolate cubes, chocolate powder, vanilla

# APPENDIX 3

## Research Results

The research I conducted was in three parts: a survey, a focus group on females, and a case study of one male.

The purpose of the survey and focus group was to analyze people's usual thoughts and behavior around food and exercise. I wanted to determine whether people who live different lifestyles could adapt to my method. I also wanted to know if diet-free people had their own tricks to stay in control of their weight, so that I could share that insight with others.

The case study gave me evidence that the method works for males as well as females.

The survey comprised 15 questions, each having detailed subsections. The information gathered was from a range of areas including personal, physical, work level and industry, water intake quantity and timing, exercise style and duration, experience with dieting, food-intake style and behavior, adaptability to change, athletic background, self-acceptance, restaurant preferences, travel, pregnancy, sleep, breathing, comments, tips, or hints relating to food.

Thanks to the Internet, the people who answered the questionnaire were from various backgrounds, ages, and 25 nationalities living in different parts of the world. The total number of respondents was 100, 50 percent were male and

50 percent were female; 79 percent were between 24 and 36 years old, most of them were fit and healthy.

During the focus group, I discussed different topics with a few women, some of whom had been pregnant in the past.

The greatest thing I discovered by interviewing others was that certain people think the same way I do when it comes to food and were using similar methods that worked for them. They were very content with their figures.

The case study involved an architect in his early forties who wanted to lose weight. I told him he looked fine, but that it would be better if he could melt one layer of fat off his body. I figured about 20 kilos (45 pounds) would be perfect. In under six months, he changed his eating habits to healthier ones, was back to working out regularly, and had fun losing the weight because of how easy this method is. He became more confident and attractive, and I was so proud of our achievement.

### *General Survey Responses Relating to Food and Lifestyle Changes:*

- 53% of people can adapt to change fast or very fast
- 75% eat what they like regularly
- 57% do not eat food that is in front of them if they are not hungry
- 31% would eat food even if they were not hungry
- 57% of people get up from the table once full
- 25% would eat a bit more and stop
- 11% would continue until super full
- 30% eat late at night
- 46% do not eat late at night
- 40% of people do not cook their own meals
- 51% cook their own meals
- 14% sleep after eating
- 22% eat less during weekdays
- 31% of people skip breakfast

- 14% skip lunch
- 9% skip dinner; the rest skip meals when not hungry or randomly
- 42% consider their food habits bad, and 58% consider their food habits good[9]
- 40% think their body is strong
- 65% of people like or love their body
- 28% do not like their body
- 85% were athletic and did some sports when younger, either basketball, volleyball, dancing, boxing, or other
- 58% gain weight quickly and 42% gain weight slowly
- 46% lose weight quickly and 48% lose weight slowly
- The most popular foods were Middle Eastern, Japanese, Chinese, and Italian
- 49% of people eat out daily, 20% once a week, 20% twice a week, 20% three times a week, and 7% eat out all week.
- 50% eat two courses, 35% eat one course, and 15% eat three courses at a restaurant
- Most people sleep six, eight, or nine hours every night
- 69% of people breathe shallowly, and 31% breathe deeply using their entire lung capacity
- 32% of the women who responded had been pregnant at some point in their lives

---

9 Good habits were always associated with eating salads, fiber, nuts, vegetables, and fruits or regularly eating three meals a day with medium portions, as well as exercising and drinking water. Bad habits were always associated with junk food, sweets, alcohol, eating late, and skipping meals daily.

# APPENDIX 4

## Comments from Survey Respondents

These comments were gathered from some of the surveys. Notice that the advice is very similar to what I have been giving throughout the book. Some are funny, and some are helpful, so I kept a bit of everything.

- Food is a blessing; do not hate yourself when you eat.
- Grilled is better than fried, fresh better than canned.
- I wish I had more time to experiment with cooking and learn more interesting dishes.
- I do not believe in food restriction, but in freedom and the capacity to listen to our bodies.
- I love to eat really great-tasting food, and I indulge in ways that used to be out of control, but recently, I have been overcoming the urges. I love to cook, so refined food is a lifestyle.
- Easy food preparation is key to motivation in maintaining a healthy diet.
- You are what you eat; carrots are good.
- I love raw food like almonds.
- Fresh foods are always better than preserved ones.
- I love to try new dishes.
- Food intake directly changes with physical activity.
- Don't eat fried food; eat healthy steamed food.

- Eat three times daily; eat fibers; do everything in moderation.
- Eat, eat, eat, and let it out!
- Food is great, but I try not to make my life revolve around it.
- Waste or waist?
- Many people confuse thirst with hunger, because the feeling in the stomach is the same.
- If you order dessert at a restaurant, share it with someone. Go for flavor in food, rather than quantity—it is often your taste buds that need to be satisfied.
- Keep smiling; no problem is ever really a big problem.
- A positive attitude reflects on all aspects of your life!
- Don't eat the food if you don't know what's in it!—unless you are *really* hungry ☺.
- Have a nice, sexy body.
- Work out and do not diet.
- Five things not to do immediately after eating: 1. Don't drink; 2. Don't smoke; 3. Don't eat dessert; 4. Don't sleep; and 5. Don't make love.
- Do your food shopping once a week, choosing healthy and easy-to-prepare meals.
- Try not to overeat when you eat out; make sure to eat salads and fruits regularly.
- Try to keep away from oily fried food as much as you can.
- A little bit of everything is usually enough; be fit and enjoy your life.
- Do what's best for *you*.
- People who like to eat are usually good listeners.
- Believe that you are the hero of the story that is your life.
- Eat only at breakfast, lunch, and dinner; do not eat between those times, especially small snacks, such as chips, cookies, etc.
- Always exercise to take toxins out of your system, and then eat fewer calories than you burn; exercise to stay lean.

- Less sugar is better, good honey is best.
- If you want to lose weight, don't deprive yourself of the foods you like. Discipline and exercise are key factors in living a healthy lifestyle.
- Water, apples, and yogurt are perfect for the body and soul.
- Work out a lot; it is medicine.
- Don't eat late.
- Do everything in moderation.
- Protein shakes and cereal are a great way to get everything you need in a meal with ultra-short prep time!
- Your body regulates itself when you exercise. At that point, food doesn't matter anymore, and your body automatically makes better choices. Even if you do eat, you don't have to feel guilty, so it brings forth positive thinking. Stop worrying about food and feeling guilty, and the weight just comes off by itself.
- People are very particular in their likes and dislikes. As far as food goes, if you are hungry, you want to eat what you like. Just be sure to check on the quantity.
- We eat to live, not live to eat.
- Eat when you are hungry.
- Your body will tell you what it needs if you understand it well.
- Life's too short, so don't diet, but do treat your body as a temple.
- I have to enjoy what I feel like eating, not think about my body too much, and acquire a taste for healthy things and good cooking.
- I believe my body is a machine capable of doing a lot more than I think; I am testing my limits.
- Do not spoil yourself too much with fancy food.
- Eat the right foods for a healthy mind and body.
- The more control you have over the amount and timing of food, the better lifestyle you live.
- Consider becoming vegetarian.

- The right amount and type of food is always what a good body is made out of.
- Do not eat more than your body needs.
- "Man shall not live by bread alone but on every work that comes from the living God" (Matthew 4:4).
- I prefer to maintain my body.
- Fruits and vegetables are essential to a healthy body.
- Eat well, sleep well, and live well.
- You are what you eat; your body reflects your past habits; you are stuck with the body you have built during your youth, but it's never too late to change.
- Food is for enjoyment and nourishment. If it is good, I eat it; if not, I don't. I don't deprive myself. I eat when I am hungry.
- I treat my body like I treat my car. You have to maintain your body so it can maintain you!
- Healthy food makes my body happy.

\* \* \*

# APPENDIX 5

## List of Headings

## Chapter 1 — Thoughts     1

# Chapter 2—Principles    45

# Chapter 3 — Texture                       **55**

# Chapter 6—Habits                                 **103**

# ACKNOWLEDGMENTS

This project was started in Dubai and completed in the United States, thanks to many people.

Thank you especially to my family and friends, whose belief in me made this achievement possible.

Thank you to those who tried some of the things I mentioned and while implementing those changes in their lives, developed fitter bodies and more self-confidence.

Thank you to the people who filled out the survey; the answers often proved to be astonishingly relevant to this book. The survey helped me to investigate and learn about people's habits pertaining to food and exercise, to gather insights they had that could be helpful for others, and to discover what they believe worked for them. I want to thank them for passing on their knowledge and tricks so that I could share them with other people.

I dedicate this book to my sister Rouba; she is the one who initiated the idea of writing a book that could help people to lose weight and live healthy ever after. She has been my greatest inspiration throughout the years. She also helped me tremendously in reviewing and editing.

Thank you to my parents, who always ate and still eat super-healthy and super-yummy food at home, exercise, and always push us in that direction.

Thank you to my mother, who learned numerous sports and taught aerobics three times a day even while pregnant with my brother. Her passion and career is art, so traveling from city to city to exhibit her Zen artworks has kept her in great shape throughout her life. Mother always encouraged us as kids to follow our dreams no matter what they were. She believed in my book, and this gave me much more confidence in myself.

Thank you to my father, who is active and enjoys hiking, skiing, diving, and traveling. He always preaches that health is one of the best forms of wealth. He also helped me a lot with editing.

Thank you to my husband, who was the first to read the manuscript and spent many nights editing the book. He loves reading, sports and travel.

Thank you to my brother, who is so particular about what he eats and drinks; he treats his body with a lot of respect.

Thank you to Georges Maroun for taking professional photos of my full workout program, those should appear on the book website.

Thank you to Lora, Barbara Wolf, Margaret Anderson, Keala Carter and Sammar Younes for their generous time in reading and reviewing the book.

Many thanks to the team at CreateSpace; they were very positive, supportive, creative, and professional throughout this project.

I dedicate this book to all the people—those I know and those I do not—who will end up looking and feeling wonderful as a result of reading and applying the knowledge in this book.

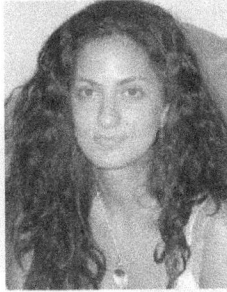

# ABOUT THE AUTHOR

Racha Zeidan is a Lebanese photographer and author raised in the United Arab Emirates. She earned her Business Management degree from London's Webster University, and worked in marketing and contemporary art in Dubai and Abu Dhabi.

As a world traveler, conscious of emerging health trends, Zeidan has become an advocate for healthy living and a coach to those seeking weight management.

She now lives with her American husband in Virginia where they enjoy hiking.

For more information please visit www.greatbodynodiet. com and www.rachazeidan.com.